BACK TO THE ROOTS
Essays on Performing Arts of India

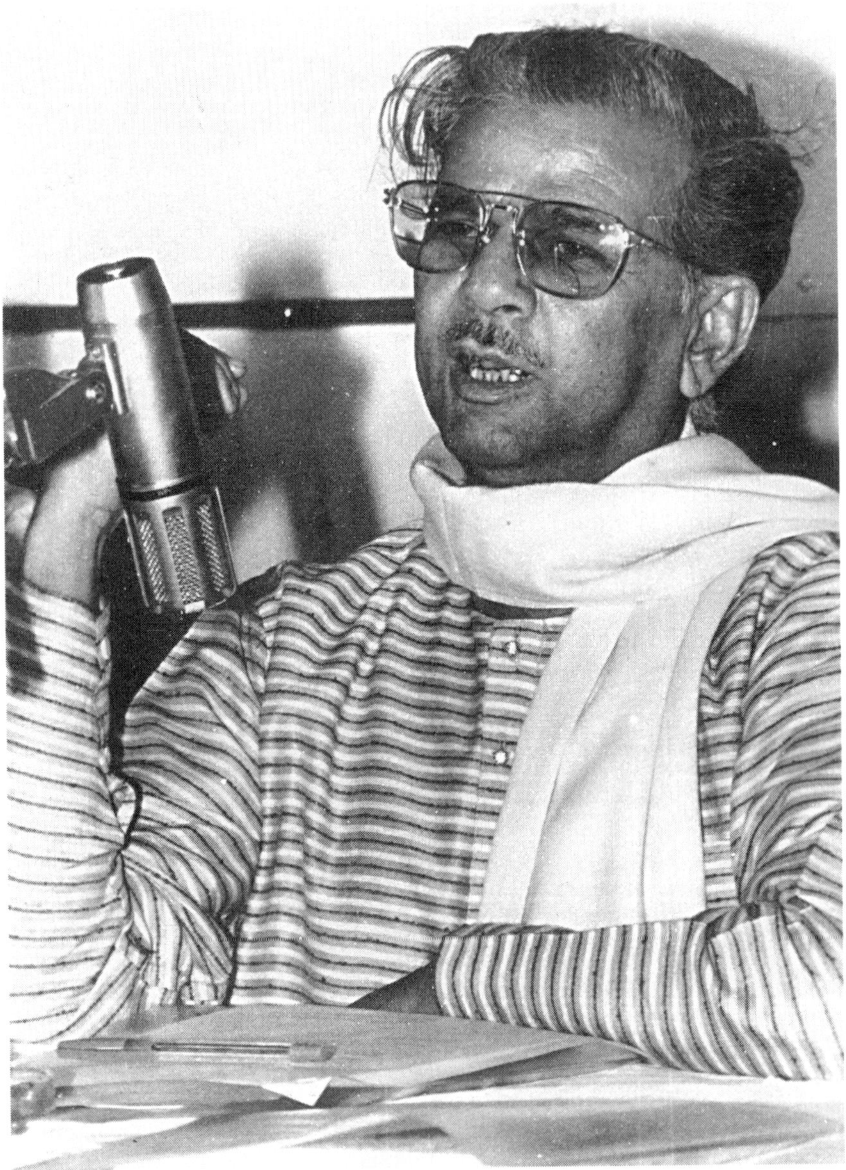

Back to the Roots

Essays on Performing Arts of India

JIWAN PANI

Compiled by
REBA PANI

Designed by
DILLIP KUMAR TRIPATHY

MANOHAR
2004

First published 2004

ISBN 81-7304-560-7

Published by
Ajay Kumar Jain for
Manohar Publishers & Distributors
4753/23 Ansari Road, Daryaganj
New Delhi 110 002

Edited by
Renuka Narayanan

Typeset by
Ajay Art, Delhi 110 085

Printed at
Lordson Publishers Pvt. Ltd.
Delhi 110 007

Contents

Illustrations

Foreword

THIS BOOK MIRRORS Jiwan Pani's multifaceted personality as a poet, lyricist, cultural commentator, research scholar, translator and an art administrator. Through his writings, he has strived to propagate and popularize Indian dance traditions. The essays in this anthology bring out his concern for the dance forms, their evolution and survival. His writings have persuasiveness and engaging quality, his language is visual and artistic that makes a reader committed. Throughout his career Jiwan Pani was after an intense pursuit to find out the *kala mula shastra*, roots of the performing art traditions.

Like the *Sutradhara* of a traditional play, he has woven the homogeneity of a tradition at the levels of *loka* and *shastriya*. For him the *loka* is a level of experience and *shastriya* is rootedness in textual erudition. He views facets of learning, *vidya*—like philosophy, linguistic, poetics dramaturgy and religion—as an alphabet to understand the Indian art traditions, be it dance, play, poetry or painting.

Delhi provided a second home to Jiwan Pani who primarily belongs to Orissa and its cultural traditions which nourished him as a poet. The liberal artistic climate of princely Baripada gave him a cosmopolitan temper to look beyond for possibilities. Jiwan Pani is intensely sensitive to the fragrance of his soil, sunsets and moonlit nights, to the cloud-laden skies and dancing peacocks, to the surging waves and the deep mystic forests. These unique life experiences emerge as poetic images, similes and metaphors. Jiwan's poetic experiences are sung by millions and he is a romantic and pastoral reality to them. In the pages of this book you can hear his authoritative intimate voice making a definite statement.

His analytic mind deals elaborately with the problem of translation. A sensitive scholar rooted in a regional tradition, Jiwan Pani feels intensely the need to find suitable terminologies which could justifiably express local *paribhasha* terms to an Indian or world audience without sacrificing their cultural imperatives. When he writes on Kalidasa and Indian dance, he wishes not to lose the poetic intensity and distort the intent of the original words. He rightly says, poetry is to be sung and poetry is to be danced.

He writes about individual experience in arts, about *rasanubhuti* as the life's culminating attainments only to make the reading of this book an experience. For the fulfilment of such a consummate experience he searches for parallels and alternatives in various dance forms of the country, beginning with Chhau in Mayurbhanj, Seraikela and Purulia, Sahi Jatra and Mughal Tamasha of Orissa, Satra dances and Bhaona theatres of Assam, and Sumagaleela of Manipur. His search for 'Vision and Resonance' lands him in strange places, he links the Shadow Puppetry and Ravanchhaya of Orissa to the Chinese, Turkish and Javanese traditions. To understand the intricate language of dance forms, he studies handicrafts and traditional ritualistic art like *kolam*, *jhoti*, *alpana* and *aripana*. He watches the foot works, hand gestures, facial expressions and bodily postures and, how like seasons, they change from Odissi to Kuchipuddi to Kathak.

He, in his research pursuits, strides into linguistics and etymological terrains to trace the connectiveness of Ravanchhaya with Javanese puppets. The Javanese word '*wanda*' transforms into '*vandha*', meaning posture or composition; the syllable *wa* becomes *ba* in Oriya leading to *bandhanritya* of Odissi, again equivalent to '*bandhaputita*'.

The reader will find this anthology handy to refer to any of the persistent cultural forms, traditions and functions like the Jagannatha cult, Indian myths, *Guru-Shishya Parampara*, *Nayaka-Nayika bheda*, Kalidasa's *Shakuntala*, Jayadeva's *Gitagovinda*, Prahlada Nataka, Kathakali and the Vedic vision of the seers.

The reader may find some overlapping across essays dealing with similar themes but varying in depth and emphasis. To retain the author's touch and sensitivity as also to capture their authenticity, the publishers have wisely refrained from editing and deleting such passages from the essays and retained them in their original form. The reader's indulgence is sought in this behalf.

Jiwan Pani's innovative persona weaves facts and philosophies, aspirations and achievements, experiences and ecstacies into this compendium. This anthology is a fitting tribute to the departed soul as well as to the Indian arts.

DINANATH PATHY

Dharma is Not Religion

INDIAN CULTURE would seem as secular right from the beginning, thousands of years ago. What is now known as Hindu religion is neither a religion nor was it named Hindu. The Vedic *munis* and *rishis* who originated it, named it Sanatana Dharma. *Sanatana* means eternal, but *dharma* cannot be translated as 'religion'. The word *dharma* has been formed from the verbal root *dhri* that means 'to hold'. Therefore, *dharma* aims at holding a person, not binding him. On the other hand 'religion' has been formed with two Latin roots: *re* which means 'again', and *ligare* which means 'to bind'. The difference between holding and binding will be clear by giving an example. Imagine that a bird fell down while it was flying, because somehow one of its wings was injured. To save the bird from being trampled, someone took the bird from the ground and held it on his open palm. The moment the injured wing heals, the bird is free to fly again. This is holding. If, however, the injured bird is kept inside a cage, it may be safe, but it cannot fly again into the sky when its injured wing gets better. This is binding. Therefore, it can be said that some home holds, prison bind. The originators of Sanatana Dharma seem to have shaped it as a way of life that is totally secular. Therefore, there is no system of conversion in this *dharma*. The concept of *dharma* is thus closer to *culture* than to religion.

It is worthwhile knowing how Sanatana Dharma came to be known as the Hindu religion. The originators of Vedic culture and Sanatana Dharma lived in the region close to the banks of the Sindhu river (Indus) and its tributaries. The first foreign invader, after Vedic culture was fully crystallized, was Darius I, of Persia (now Iran). In the Persian language, 's' is often pronounced as 'h'. Therefore, the Sindhu became the Hindu river, and the people who were residing near its banks, the Hindus. The inscription on the tomb of Darius at Persepolis calls the people living near the Sindhu river the Hindus Duries. The Persians annexed a portion of the region around the Sindhu river during the later part of sixth century BC. The next foreign invader in this region was Alexander of Greece during the later part of the fourth century BC. His incursion into India was through Persia and therefore he came to know the people living in the region around the Sindhu river as 'Hindu'. In Greek however, 'h' is pronounced softly. The Greeks called the 'Hindu' the Indus and the land, India. Thus our country Bharat came to be known as India in the West. Both Hindu and India are historical misnomers which continue two millennia later!

The originators of the Vedic culture shaped Sanatana Dharma in such a way that the followers of this way of life would aim at living at a higher plane of consciousness. Deep meditation gave them the insight that an individual and the vast cosmos have an intense relationship. This relationship can only be realized at a much higher level of consciousness. For this they devised two methods, *yoga* and *puja*. *Yoga* although a much superior method, is not easy for the common man. *Puja*, on the other hand, is a much easier method as it is done in a symbolic manner. What is performed at the time of *puja* is called a ritual. To modern thinkers, rituals appear in a completely different perspective. Joseph

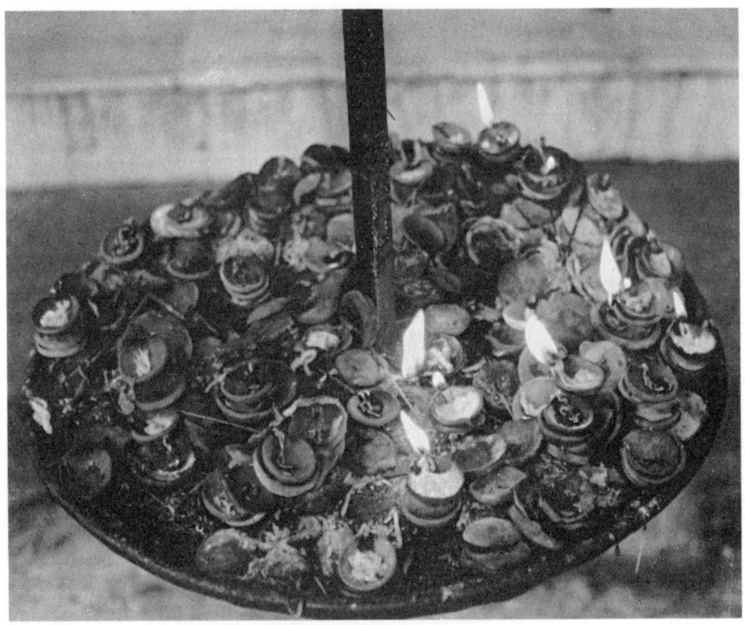

1. *Ghee* lamps, the symbol of sacredness.
Photo: Dillip Tripathy.

Campbell says, 'Ritual can be defined as an enactment of a myth. By participating in a ritual, you are actually experiencing a mythological life. And it's out of that participation that one can learn to live spiritually.' Behind each of our rituals there is a myth and if that myth is not taken into account then the ritual appears as empty religious activity.

Let us take the *puja* ritual of placing a pot, usually earthen, filled with water, in which a small branch of mango leaves is dipped and over which a coconut is kept. This is called *mangala kalasha* meaning the 'auspicious pot'. It is a focus of prayer and worship during certain *pujas*. Its symbolism is as deep as poetic.

In Indian philosophy the ultimate being is *Brahma* who is beyond time and space, has no shape, and contains the whole cosmos within him. A human being, on the other hand, is finite and bound by time cannot intellectually grasp *Brahma* that is infinite and eternal. But he or she can experience it momentarily deep within one's self if the state of the mind is elevated to a height beyond the gravitation of the intellect. The main aim of a *puja* is to glimpse *Brahma* deep within oneself. The fragile earthen pot symbolises the perishable physical body of the person performing the *puja*. The water inside the pot is the symbol of life. The symbolism of the mango leaves is really poetic. A person experiences both happiness and sorrow throughout life. While happiness is sweet, sorrow is sour. The mango is a fruit that has both sweetness and sourness in such a way that the latter does not combat the former, but enhances it. Therefore, the mango leaves symbolize a state of mind in the worshipper who, at the time of *puja* site to prays with the awareness that the sorrows of life do not eclipse happiness, but rather enhance it. With such a buoyant and aspiring state of mind, the worshipper goes forward to do the *puja*. The symbolism of the coconut is both poetic and metaphysical. There are several layers that separate one from the experience of *Brahma*. The different layers of the coconut represents them. The outermost layer, which is shining green or yellow-green symbolizes the reality that our five senses experience. The next layer is tough fibres that represent superstitions and blind faith. Beyond that is the hard shell of the coconut. This is the symbol of Ego. When one goes beyond it, the white kernel of the coconut is reached, that symbolizes Divinity. The next 'layer' is water that is the symbol of the beginning of creation. Beyond the water, is an empty space filled with the aroma of the coconut. This symbolizes the *Brahma* that is philosophically defined as a nothingness that contains everything. The *mangala kalasha* is thus a symbolic expression of a mortal and finite human being, aspiring for an experience of *Brahma.*

From the ritual of breaking a coconut as an auspicious beginning, it is clear that the worshipper symbolically says that he/she is prepared to tear apart all the layers that separate him/her from the experience of *Brahma.* Thus when the myth and symbolism behind our rituals are considered, they are no longer 'religious' activities but entirely secular, like an allegorical poem with universal meaning.

Yajna for the Eyes

KALIDASA, THE GREAT Sanskrit poet and playwright, in his play *Malavikaagnimitram*, says, 'Sages look upon dance as the *yajna* that is pleasing to the eyes of gods (*deva*)'. *Devanam idam amananti munayah kantam kratum chakyasham*. The implications of this succinct statement are as deep as it is extensive. The two key words *yajna* and *deva* are full of subtle nuances, which if rightly understood, the doors will open to a fuller appreciation of the aesthetic quality of the various styles of Indian art dances.

Yajna is translated into English as 'sacrifice', which is not an apt translation, because *yajna* has been formed from the verbal root *yaj* which means 'to worship'. In many kinds of *yajna*, animal sacrifice is not a must. In any kind of *yajna*, however, the ritual of offering several ladlefuls of *ghee* (clarified butter) to the burning fire is performed. The ritual has a very deep and metaphysical symbolism. Thinkers today view ritual from a completely different perspective. Joseph Campbell says, 'Ritual can be defined as an enactment of a myth. By participating in a ritual, you are actually experiencing a mythological life. And it's out of that participation that one can learn to live spiritually.' Notions about mythology have also undergone a complete change. No longer are myths considered as sheer figments of imagination. Today the opinion is that myths, poetical metaphors and symbols have always been used whenever someone has tried to express innermost experiences which ordinary language or plain words cannot convey. Mythological characters are like masks behind which we may see the multiple faces of our complex life. *Yajna* has a myth behind it and the ritual of offering *ghee* to the fire is steeped in symbolism.

The myth associated with *yajna* is the *Shatapatha Brahma* a Vedic literature of great antiquity. The succinct expression, if elaborated, will be as follows:

The first *yajna* was performed by the *Prajapati*, the creator who dismembered his body into countless parts and strewed them all over space. Thus the Universe was created like a jigsaw puzzle. The main aim of the *yajna* performed by a human being is to re-assemble mentally the scattered Universe, partly, if not whole, so that the unity in diversity is fully comprehended.

Thus *yajna* is a meditative worship through symbolic enactment, i.e. rituals. One of the very important *yajnas* is *Ashvamedha*, in which a horse is sacrificed. The horse is a powerful symbol of the ultimate divinity. The *Brihadaranyaka Upanishad* begins with the description of the sacrificial horse. Going through the description one will be convinced that the horse sacrificed in the *yajna* is but a symbol. The English translation of the passage in Sanskrit is as follows:

The head of the sacrificial horse verify the dawn. The eye of the sacrificial horse is the sun; the vital force, the air; the open mouth the fire named *Vaishvanara*, the trunk, the year; the back is heaven, the belly the sky; the hoof the earth; the flanks the four directions; the ribs the intermediate directions; the limbs the seasons; the joints the months and fortnights; the bones the stars; the feet the day and night; the flesh the clouds; the half-digested food the sands; the arteries and the veins the rivers; the liver and spleen the mountains; the hairs the herbs and trees; the forepart the rising sun. Its yawn is lightning, its shaking the body is thunder, its making water is rain, its neighing is indeed speed.

This highly poetic and metaphysical symbolism is for meditation, by the person who is to perform the *Ashvamedha yajna.* When the meditation goes to a deeper state, the sacrificial horse is identified with *Prajapati* the cosmic being. Then the horse is sacrificed as *Prajapati* did to create the Universe. Only kings were permitted to do the *yajna* with

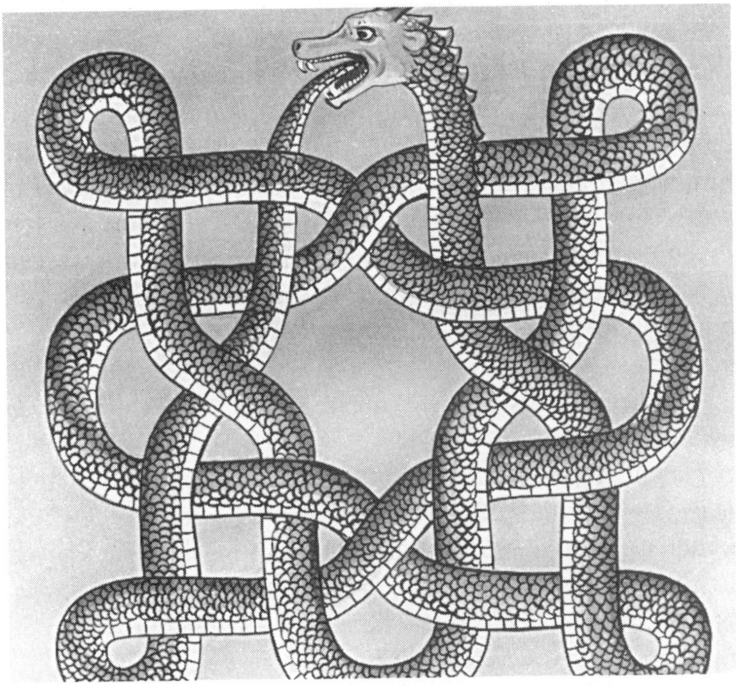

2. A Naga Mandal with a dragon head.
Photo: Sangeet Natak Akademi (SNA), New Delhi

horse sacrifice. Any other person had to meditate on his own body as that of the sacrificial horse described in the Upanishad. At the end of the meditation he was to imagine that he was dismembering his body and strewing it all around space.

The ritual of pouring ladlefuls of clarified butter on the flaming fire is also steeped in highly poetic symbolism. In Indian mythology, milk symbolizes human awareness. Lord Vishnu who sustains the entire creation, has been conceived as reclining on the surface of the vast ocean of milk. The being that sustains the entire Universe can never be finite like a human being. The human form in which Vishnu has been conceived is the *moorti* that literally means the concretized form of one who is abstract. The abstract Vishnu cannot be perceived by the five senses of a human being. His presence can only be experienced in the awareness. Therefore, Lord Vishnu is depicted as reclining on the ocean of milk. Again, *Kshira Sagara Manthana*, the Churning of the Ocean of Milk, is a well-known episode from Indian mythology. When the

Ocean of Milk was churned many beautiful and beneficial things like *amrit* (ambrosia of immortality) came out of the sea together with deadly poison called *halahal*. The poison could have destroyed the world, had not Lord Shiva, the ultimate *yogi*, swallowed it. This happens when human awareness and intelligence is churned. The churning has given us many arts, medicines, that are beneficial to us but it has also produced nuclear weapons, the *halahal* to contain which tremendous effort is being made.

When milk is churned, butter comes out. When human awareness is churned, love, affection and other nobler emotions come out. That is why Krishna, the incarnation of total love, is so fond of butter. When butter is heated, *ghee*, the clarified butter, is produced. When the nobler sentiments are subjected to *tapasya*, the consciousness is clarified. The root of *tapasya* is 'tap', which means heat. Therefore, *ghee* that is poured on the flaming fire symbolizes clarified awareness.

The flame of the fire of which the clarified butter is offered is another powerful symbol in Indian mythology. Among the Vedic gods, Agni, the fire god, is the leader. Agni literally means that which goes upward. Fire is the only thing in the world that goes upward, acting against the gravitation but without leaving the plane of its origin. Balloons do go upward but they all leave the place of their origin. The fire, therefore, symbolizes that kind of human aspiration which goes up towards spiritualism without leaving the wordly existence. In a *yajna*, such an aspiration is offered the clarified consciousness.

Deva is the other key word according to Kalidasa. Although *deva* or *devata* generally means a god, the literal meaning reveals the Indian concept of God. The verbal root of *deva* or *devata* is *div* that means 'to shine' or 'to brighten'. The day in Sanskrit, as also in many regional languages, is *diva* whose root is *div*. When the darkness of the night is dispelled, it becomes bright. Therefore the day is called *diva*. Since the root of *deva* is *div*, it literally means 'shining being'. If the being is conceived as having feminine quality, she is called a *devi*. There is a synonym of *deva*. It is *sura*, having the root *sur* that also means 'bright'. The domain where these shining beings live is called *svarga* (equivalent to heaven) having the root *svar* which again means 'bright'. The being who is not shining and emits darkness is called *asura*. The prefix 'a' means 'not'. In Indian mythology the *asuras* are demonic titans. Nobler attributes are considered bright and baser, non-bright. According to Indian thinking it is the *ahankara* (ego) which imparts baser qualities to human beings. Therefore, whether it is *yoga* or *puja* (worship) the main aim is to discard ego. The *devas* are shining beings because they are totally devoid of ego. Indian mythology is full of wars between *devas* and *asuras*. When the *devas* acquire some amount of ego they are defeated by the *asuras* and the domain of *svarga* comes under the rule of the *asuras*. When the *devas* realize their fault and totally discard ego, they defeat the *asuras* and regain their domain of *svarga*. When a human being is full of nobler qualities and is not the least egotistic, that person is identified with a *deva* or *devi*, as the case may be.

According to Indian aestheticians, it is necessary for a person to suspend his/her ego while watching the performance of an art dance, because ego tends to fetter the person to the everyday realities which may cloud his/her aesthetic experience.

According to Kalidasa, the dancer while dancing, performs a *yajna*. *Yajna*, as just discussed, is basically a meditation to experience the ultimate divinity through rituals. In case of the performance of dance, the dancing itself is both meditation and ritual. That is why perhaps performance of Indian dances appears to have ritualistic overtones. As said earlier, the main aim of either a *yajna* or a *puja* is to experience the ultimate divinity. When the ultimate divinity is charged with the urge to create, it is qualified as *Prajapati*. Before it stirs with the urge to create, the being is non-qualifiable. This state of ultimate reality/divinity is named as *Brahma* which, according to Indian philosophy, is the only being. All the created things, including the human beings, are *becomings*. Sri Aurobindo has given a wonderful analogy of the sea and waves to explain the relationship of the being and the becoming. If the sea is the being, the waves are *becomings*. The waves are not separate from the sea. They are only different states of the sea. They rise from the sea and merge into the sea. We call them waves as if they were separate from the sea. The sea becomes the waves. Therefore, they are only *becomings*. Similarly, it is from *Brahma* that all things rise to become what they are and they merge again into *Brahma*. It is the force of *maya* that makes us think a becoming is a being. *Maya* is, therefore, neither illusion nor hallucination, its nearest English translation is perhaps 'relative reality'.

When the *Brahma* is engaged in creation, it becomes qualified as *Prajapati*, which state is known in Indian philosophy as *Saguna Brahma* and when it is non qualifiable, that state is *Nirguna Brahma*. The highest aspiration of an Indian worshipper is to experience the *Nirguna Brahma*, who is formless and beyond time and space. To experience it is not at all easy. Through long and immense *yogic* meditation, one can, however momentarily experience the *Nirguna Brahma*.

Indian philosophers and aestheticians were of opinion that since aesthetic experience is characterized by the immersion of the subject in the aesthetic object to the exclusion of all else, this momentary interruption of everyday life is akin to the beatitude of ecstasy or the experience of *Brahma*.

Bhatta Nayak, a philosopher and aesthetician of the ninth century says, 'This aesthetic pleasure is poured forth spontaneoulsy by the word, like a cow, for love of her children, for this reason it is different from that which is (laboriously) milked by *yogins*.'

According to Bhatta Nayak, the experience of *Brahma* by the artist and by the *yogin* differ slightly, because to the former it comes spontaneously, whereas the latter has to make a good deal of effort through arduous *yogic* practices. Later aestheticians echoed what Bhatta Nayak said, that the two kinds of the experience of *Brahma* are like twins. It may therefore be said that the *yajna* of dance is twin to the regular kinds of *yajnas*.

Kalidasa says that the dance is pleasing to the eyes of the *devas*. Here *deva* does not mean the mythical shining beings who are conceived as residing in *svarga* (domain of light) but those among the audience who have nobler sentiments and have suspended their ego for watching the performance of a dance.

Before the dance proper begins, the accompanying musicians and the dancer go through some preliminaries known as *poorva-ranga*. These preliminaries aim at *sadharani karana* which mean generalization, or impersonalization.

The *poorva-ranga* aimed at *sadharani karana* may not be effective for a person in the audience who unlike a *deva* is not ready to suspend his/her ego. As a result the person cannot break away from the moorings of everyday life that is limited by time and space.

The analysis of Kalidasa's statement thus leads to the conclusion that in order to enjoy the aesthetic experience provided by Indian dances, the spectator should qualify to be *deva* like, who in Indian aesthetics is known as *sahridaya darshaka*, meaning a spectator vibrating on the same frequency as that of the dancers. There are four kinds of spectators. The *darshaka*, an ordinary spectator who comes seeking entertainment, usually not rising above the physicality of the dancer. Then comes the *sahridaya darshaka*, who wants the pleasure of aesthetic experience. The *rasika* is a connoisseur who not only enjoys the aesthetic experience but also makes an assessment of the proficiency of the dancer and to what degree he/she has been successful in giving the audience aesthetic experience. The *prashnika* is an acknowledged expert of dance who can give his considered opinion on the techniques of dance, should some kind of controversy crop up. The minimum requirement for being a *qualified* spectator of Indian art dance, is to be a *sahridaya darshaka*.

The Doctrine of *Natya*

ALTHOUGH *NATYA* means theatre, it used to connote in ancient India something much more than a mere theatrical performance. At present, theatre serves either as a form of entertainment or as a tool for reformation. The theatre with such motive is quite prone to degeneration, especially when the performers are professional. The theatre that aims at entertaining the audience may degenerate into a cheap and sloppy show for popular appeal whereas that aiming at social change may result in pure propaganda. However, the ancient Indian exponents of the theatre conceived *natya* as a powerful means for deepening our comprehension of the infinite complexities of human life.

Again, it is significant, India regarded theatre as the focal point of all arts. It was not an arbitrary perspective, but a well-reasoned one, since theatre is the only branch of art that has the potential to incorporate various forms of arts, crafts and even technology. This is quite clear when Bharata Muni says in the *Natya Shastra*, 'There is no such knowledge, no such craft, no such education, no such art, no such *yoga*, no such activity, which cannot be seen in *natya*.' Therefore, in ancient India *natya* was regarded as the fifth Veda which literally means a deep knowledge.

According to the *Natya Shastra* written about two thousand years ago and which down the centuries, has been the most authoritative grammar for various artistic expressions including poetry, *natya* can admirably blend all the different kinds of *yoga*. If one does not understand what *yoga* actually means, one can neither have a clear idea of *natya* nor have any understanding of Indian culture.

Yoga literally means union. In Indian philosophy it means the process of purifying consciousness in such a way that the nature of the underlying soul (*purusa*) becomes apparent. As a result, one sees the essential otherness of soul from material nature, thereby gaining release from bondage to the latter. Consciousness thus released, finds that thought and its object are inseparably united. The dichotomy between subject and object becomes irrelevant. The total union of the objective perspective with that of the subjective is, in fact one of the results of *yoga*.

In order to comprehend the concept of *natya* another word has to be rightly understood. That is *yajna*. It is not merely a symbolic ritual where clarified butter (*ghrita*, i.e. *ghee*) is poured on the fire burning on a sanctified altar. Its import is far deeper. There is a fascinating myth in *Shatapatha Brahma*, which may serve as a key to our understanding what *yajna* connotes:

Prajapati, the Lord of Creatures, offered himself in sacrifice (*yajna*). He thus dismembered himself. All those separated limbs and faculties formed the universe—all that exists from the gods down to the smallest particle of inert matter. It required a new and ever new sacrifice to build the dismembered *Prajapati* up again and again, and renew the universe, and thus keep up the uninterrupted revolution of time and matter. The *Shatapatha Brahma* says, '*Prajapati's* eyes swelled, they fell out, then the *ashva* was produced. . . . By means of *Ashvamedha yajna* the gods restore it to its place; and verily he who performs *Ashvamedha yajna* makes *Prajapati* complete.'

Here *ashva* does not mean a horse. The root of the word is *ash* which literally means to pervade. And *medha* means-the essence. Therefore, *ashvamedha* here actually means 'the essence of pervasiveness'. For what can be more pervasive than the eyes?

Prajapati performed, the first *yajna* when he divided himself into many for creating the Universe. Each dismembered part acquired a kind of individuality. Unless sacrificed in a *yajna*, the whole could not be built up. Unless one comprehends the *whole*, one cannot have any idea of the total Truth.

Every action has an equal and opposite reaction. It is a cosmic separative force that dispersed the dismembered parts of *Prajapati*. The moment when the separative force became active, the opposite, i.e. the unifying force, was automatically created. The separative force is known as Ego, whereas the unifying force is Love. One of the main objectives of *yajna* is to consume the Ego with the assistance of clarified consciousness which is symbolized by *ghrita* in the ritual *yajna*.

As there are many systems of *yoga*, there are many forms of *yajna* too. *Natya* is that form of *yajna* which aims at consuming the terrestrial ego and restoring the terrestrial limbs of *Prajapati*. It has an intense terrestrial character which is evident from the legend of the origin of *natya* described in the very first chapter of the *Natya Shastra*.

Legend has it that in the *Tretayuga* when the morality of human beings touched the bottom of degradation, Indra, the god of gods, approached Brahma, the creative aspect of the divinity, to create something for the unpliftment of man. Brahma resorted to *yoga* and shaped the *Natya-veda* which he offered to Indra saying, 'Pass it on to those gods who are skilful, learned, bold in speech, and inured to hard work.' Indra with folded hands replied, 'O best and holy one, gods are neither able to receive and maintain it, nor are they fit to understand and make use of it.' Brahma appreciated Indra's observation and calling Bharata Muni, gave the *Natya-veda* to him for putting it to proper use.

If the above legend is analysed it will be clear that *natya* has such an intense terrestrial significance that the gods who are non-evolutionary cannot perform it. The terrestrial *yajna* symbolizes the aspiration of darkness to be transformed into light. *Natya* thus being a form of the terrestrial *yajna* aims at seeking and finding the essence behind the perceptual reality. This is precisely what any genuine work of art aims at. Therefore, perhaps Picasso defined art as a lie that makes us realize the truth. The 'truth' is obviously not the phenomenal reality but the essence behind it.

In order to understand a thing better, it is at times necessary to magnify it. If the degree of magnification is very high, the image may appear totally diferent from the physical reality. *Natya* basically aims at presenting the artistic reality of the larger than life truth. Therefore, a theatrical presentation following the concept of *natya* appears more or less non-realistic and often highly stylized.

To the sensitive, compared to such a highly stylized theatre, the dialogue-dominated 'realistic' theatre appears emaciated, peripheral and crawling. The fiery French poet and theatre prophet Antonine Artaud, therefore, described the dialogue-centred realistic theatre of the West as a theatre 'for antipoets, positivists, grammarians, grocers, and madmen'. On the other hand, the stylized Oriental theatre appeared to him 'religious', integral, metaphysical, and sensuous.

Like a religious ritual, stylized theatre very often is at the meeting point where human and non-human, meaning and chaos, finite and infinite, come together. It has the potentiality to be the theatre of the inner eye and of the outer eye at the same time. Hence, breaking loose from the moorings that bind us to the workaday reality, it presents both the visible and the invisible forms of reality, since it does sing the un-heard melody. In a stylized theatre the dance like movements and gestures of the actors, their fantastic costumes, elaborate non-realistic make up, towering headgear, all serve as symbols. And as symbols, they are vague, only pointing the way to some absolute or secret reality.

Dance is the most important of the dramatic expressions in the *natya* style. The *Harivamsa*, an important Purana of around the fourth century BC says, *natakam nanartu* which means 'a play should be danced'. Elements of dance impart to the art of acting a rare mimetic and choreographic character.

The plays for the *natya* theatre were written in Sanskrit. That is why it cannot be called Sanskrit theatre, but basically Indian theatre. The tradition of the Sanskrit theatre unfortunately got extinct by the later part of the nineteenth century except in Kutiyattam in Kerala, but the *natya* style still survives in many forms of traditional regional theatre.

Rasa in Kathak

As in other Indian classical dance styles the *abhinaya* passages in Kathak are mostly based on sung poetic lines. Often each word of the song is visually integrated through hand gestures and appropriate body movements. In Kathak, this occurs when the expressional passages are based on a *thumri* or a *bhajan* or a *ghazal.* There are however many expressional passages in the Kathak tradition, which are not based on any verbal material. The likes of *gat-nikas* and *gat-bhav* are not in any other classical dance traditions (expression through footwork).

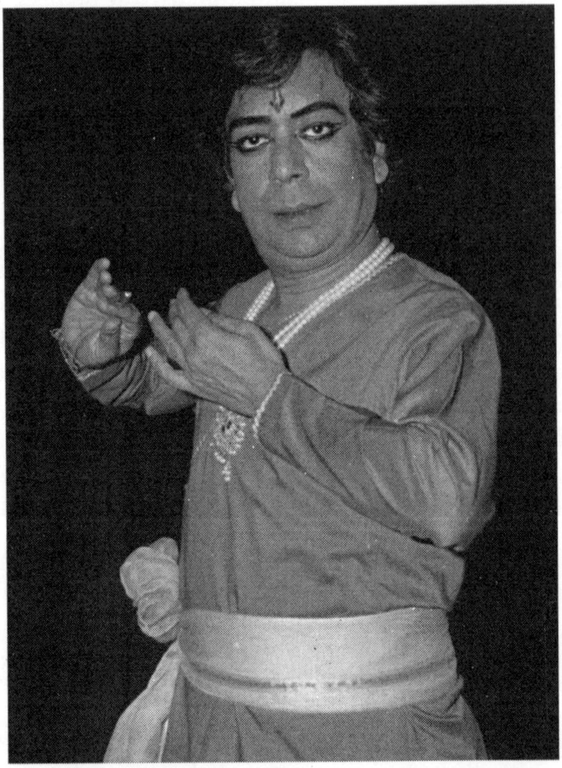

3. Birju Maharaj, famous Kathak dancer of India. Photo: SNA, New Delhi.

I am, therefore, of the opinion that the *bhavabhinaya* of Kathak can be basically categorized into three: *padabhinaya, bhav-dikhana* and *bhav-batana. Padabhinaya* is that *abhinaya* item which is based on sung poetic lines, as is found in any other dance style. But *bhav-dikhana* and *bhav-batana*, both unique aspects of Kathak, requires elaboration.

Bhav-dikhana passages are those which do not have any *vachika* (spoken) element. *Gat-nikas* and *gat-bhav* come under this category. While the pure *angikabhinaya* (body expression) of *gat-bhav* is narrative; that of *gat-nikas* is symbolic and terse. Both aim at distilling beauty and from ordinary day-to-day activities.

Guru-Shishya Parampara

DURING THE LAST few decades Indian classical dances and the dancers have been steadily, though gradually, regaining their lost social respectability. The interest of the sophisticated and educated is also increasing. Therefore, one often hears the phrase *guru-shishya parampara* being uttered, especially in the field of Indian classical dance and music. Very few however understand the depth of the concept behind it. *Guru-shishya parampara* is not merely a methodology of teaching, although the phrase seems to indicate only a personalized method of teaching.

There are basically two kinds of teaching methodology, the personalized and the impersonalized. The former is *guru-shishya parampara* and the latter is classroom teaching. Indian classical music and dance cannot be properly taught in a classroom situation. The teacher has to give personalized attention to the progress of each person taught. Therefore, *guru-shishya parampara*, even in its rudimentary form, has to be adopted. If the tradition is continued without the spirit behind it, the teaching becomes bland and the learning becomes mechanical. This is the current status of dance teaching. The situation will improve much if both the *guru* and the *shishya* understand the depth and subtlety of the teaching tradition.

The 'guru' is not really the Sanskrit equivalent of the English word 'teacher'. If the subtle difference in the meaning of the three words—teacher, *shikshak* and *guru*—is considered, the concept of *guru* will be clear. Presently, in India, a teacher in a school or a college is required to load a student

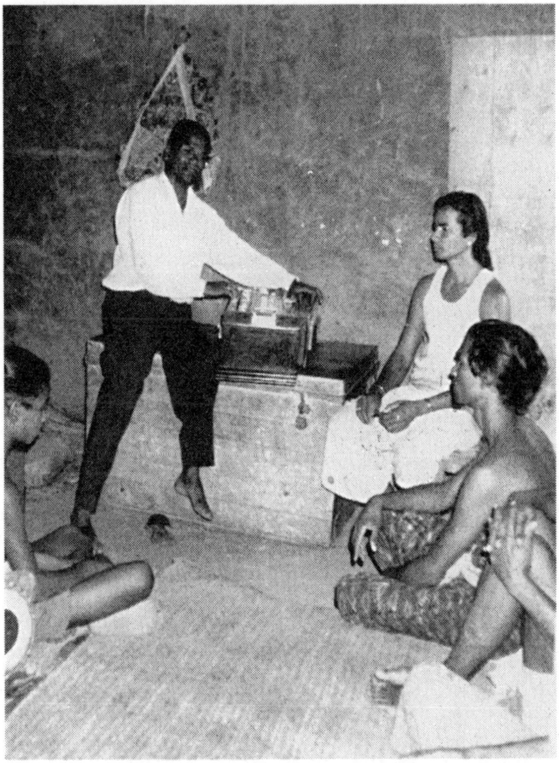

4. Biswa Bihari Khadanga (on harmonium), Prahlada Nataka director along with the performers inside the rehearsal hall, Gopinathpur village, Bhajanagar, Orissa. Photo: Dillip Tripathy.

with relevant and meaningful information which may or may not settle down as knowledge. According to traditional Indian thinking, the duty of a *shikshak* is to see that whatever he teaches is stored in the *shishya* as knowledge. The *guru* has an added responsibility. He not only imparts knowledge but also builds up personality in a student, which is coherent with his/her *swadharma*. Here *dharma* does not at all mean religion but the inherent propensity and aptitude. It is therefore a very heavy responsibility, which the *guru* bears on his capable shoulders. Unless one is a *rishi* one cannot become an accomplished *guru*. Therefore we find that all the *gurus* mentioned in our mythology and ancient literature are basically *rishis*. And a *rishi* is not merely a wise man with a flowing white beard. He is simultaneously a *yogi* and a seer. The word is derived from the Sanskrit *rish*, which means to move or to push. The definition of a *rishi* is *yah rishati gyanena samsara parum*. It means 'he who through knowledge moves or pushes the awareness beyond the phenomenal reality'. It suggests that a *rishi* has an intuitive mind and can make others capable to see beyond this relative reality of the world. A *guru*, if he is a *rishi* also, is capable of taking the awareness of the disciple to a height from where intelligence can soar towards intuition. If he/she is a *guru* of dance the disciples will feel deep within that the dance enables them to conquer the body—and then it is forgotten. But if dance is meant merely to entertain others, the body is not compared but capitalized on, not forgotten but remembered in every curve. The moment the dancer conquers and forgets the body, he/she realizes deep within that the body is now a beautifully rhythmic receptacle for the superhuman power of the soul and that all super-mundane and *true* motion—is dance.

Many a dancer, at times, begins the recital with the *guru vandana* eulogizing the guru. It says:

Gurur-brahma gurur-vishnu gurur devo maheshwarah guruh sakshat parabrahma tasmei shri guruve namah.

The *guru* is Brahma, the *guru* is Vishnu, the *guru* is Maheshwar. The *guru*, who is the incarnation of Parabrahma, to him I make my obeisance.

On the surface it may appear that the eulogy for the *guru* is highly exaggerated, but if the symbolism is understood, the concept behind it will be clear. In Indian mythology, Brahma is the creator. The guru is also a creator since he creates a new personality in the disciple. Vishnu is the divinity that sustains what has been created. The *guru* too, does that. He sees to it that the new personality created in the disciple is lasting and does not deteriorate. Maheshwar is the divinity of transformation. It is wrong to consider him as the god of annihilation or dissolution. Traditional Indian thinking asserted again and again that nothing can be annihilated, but is merely transformed. Even death is not annihilation but transformation. Maheshwar thus transforms all those who are not divine. So also a *guru* transforms all the shortcomings of a disciple into assets. The concept of Parabrahma, however, is very complex. It is conceived as a formless, all-pervading existence, beyond space and time and from it all existence comes out. In the case of the *guru*, he should have such a personality as well as such qualities that even when he is physically far away from a disciple, his presence is felt deep within. The disciple gets intuitional guidance from the *guru* even if he is not physically present near him or her.

If the dance *guru* is only a master of techniques and has no or very little idea about the various aspects and concepts connected with the dance tradition, he/she can at best be a teacher, certainly not a *guru*.

Many of those who are now imparting training in dance do not take adequate interest in the theories connected with classical dance. They think that dance is entirely a practical and applied art and has little to do with theory. Such persons perhaps do not know that in this country aesthetic thinking began with a dance guru. His name is Bharata Muni, the author of the masterly *Natya Shastra*. The *rasa* theory propounded by him is one of the infinitely subtle aesthetic theories. The kind of dance and theatre he envisaged appear ultra modern even now. The *natyadharmi* presentational technique of Bharata Muni parallels the Brechtian concept of alternation. Bharata Muni was at once a dance *guru* and a superb aesthetician. This is an ideal combination, though rare. The dance *guru* may not be an aesthetician, but he cannot afford to be ignorant about aesthetics, because the main aim of a classical dance recital is to give the audience an experience of *rasa* (aesthetic relish).

Any learning situation is graphically represented by an inverted triangle. The downward pointing apex, represents the learner (*shishya*). The learner is free to choose a *guru* who occupies the left end point of an upward-facing base. The relevant textbooks/treatises (*shastras*) occupy the right end point. The guru has to be strictly in conformity with the *shastras*. Otherwise the learning situation will be shrouded

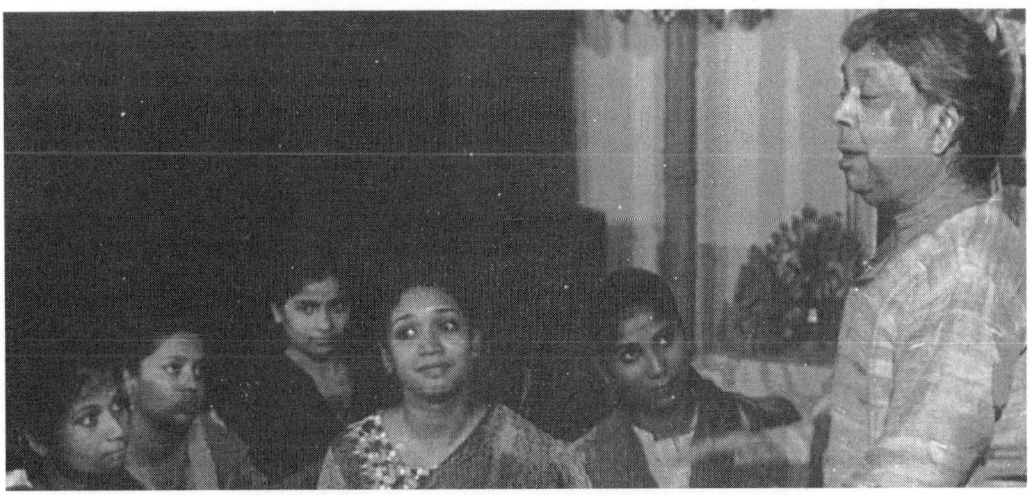

5. *Guru and Shishyas:* Birju Maharaj along with his students. Photo: SNA, New Delhi.

in confusion. The first responsibility of the *guru* is to correctly interpret the *shastras* and then see that the knowledge acquired is appropriately applied. Application should follow the acquisition of knowledge, not precede it. When application precedes acquisition of knowledge, it becomes craft. Dance when reduced to craft becomes at best a graceful parade. A genuine *guru* will never allow his/her disciples to parade a dance. Nothing can be more criminal in a *guru*. How then can a dance *guru* afford to be ignorant of the *shastras*? For the *shishyas* it is absolutely necessary to consult the *shastras* to deepen their comprehension. If the present-day dance *gurus* are not educated enough to comprehend and to rightly interpret the *shastras*, then what will befall their pupils?

The *Rasa* Theory

THE SIXTH CHAPTER of *Natya Shastra* dealing with the *rasa* is primarily for the lovers and connoisseurs of art, dance and theatre, since they experience aesthetic relish while experiencing these forms. The seventh chapter deals with the *bhavas*. This chapter is primarily for the dancer/actor, whose presentation of *bhavas*, bestows this relish on sensitive spectators.

In the *rasa* theory, *bhava* is as important as *rasa*, if not more. The word *bhava*, like myriad other words, has several meanings, The *Sanskrit-English Dictionary* by V.S. Apte lists 29 different meanings of *bhava*. Therefore, Bharata Muni, a sage and seer par excellence, to dispel any confusion, at the very beginning of the chapter, clearly indicated the right meaning of *bhava* that is used as a technical term in the aesthetic theory. He accepts the etymological meaning of the word. *Bhava* is derived from the verbal root *bhoo* that means 'to bring something into being' or 'to be born'. Therefore, *bhava* means that which brings something into being or causes something to be remembered. The aestheticians who came after Bharata Muni, give an excellent analogy to elaborate the meaning of *bhava*. Suppose you have a lump of *kasturi* (camphor) at home. While going out, you rubbed it on your kerchief. Away from home where the *kasturi* is kept, whenever you bring the kerchief near your nose you will feel as if the *kasturi* was before you or it makes you remember the lump of *kasturi* at home. The kerchief is then not the *kasturi* but the *bhava* of *kasturi*. The kerchief *evokes kasturi* before you. Therefore, *bhava* in our aesthetics means a kind of aesthetic *evocation*. In the performing arts, it is an enactment that evokes either a mood, or a thing, or an ambiance.

Everything in the area of performance, be it a stage or an arena, is the *bhava* of something. In a play when Goddess Durga kills the demon Mahishasura, the actress (*bhava* of Durga) does not actually kill the actor (*bhava* of Mahishasura), but enacts the *bhava* of killing. The enactment area thus presents a world of *bhavas*.

According to the *Natya Shastra*, there are two worlds *svabhava jagat* and *vibhava jagat*. While the former is the God-created world, the latter is the poet-created world. When Keats says, 'Heard melodies are sweet and those unheard are sweeter', he describes his experience of the *vibhava* world. Because in the *svabhava jagat* if one has not heard the melody how can it be compared to the heard melodies and said to be the sweeter? According to the logic of the *svabhava jagat* it is quite illogical! The logic of the *vibhava jagat* is totally different. In the *vibhava jagat*, it is possible that a demonic titan like Ravana has ten heads and twenty hands, which is impossible in the *svabhava jagat*. The enactment area, according to Indian aesthetics, should present primarily the *vibhava jagat*. The material for the *vibhava jagat* is taken from the *svabhava jagat* and transformed, just as the raw taste of vegetables is transformed when prepared as curry. Bharata Muni therefore analogizes the tasting of *rasa* to the tasting of curry (*vyanjana*). According to Indian aesthetics, the experience of our five sense organs of everything of the *svabhava jagat* is called *loukika anubhooti*. Raw vegetables, when eaten uncooked, give us their *loukika* taste. When cooked as curry, the culinary art transforms their *loukika* taste into *aloukika* (supernatural). Similarly, the performing art should transform all *loukika* into *aloukika*. The raw taste of some vegetables like bitter gourd (*karela*) is not pleasant to the tongue, but others like cucumber or tomato are pleasant also when uncooked. We prepare *salads* with such vegetables which though they retain their *loukika* taste are pleasant to the palate. Similarly, in the performing arts some *bhavas* like *hasya* (laughter) may retain their *loukika* expression and yet be aesthetic. This is not the case with *jugupsa* or disgust. The *bhavas* which retain their *loukika* expression are *lokadharmi* and those which are transformed into *aloukika*, spiced with elements of music, dance and costume are *natyadharmi*.

We react to everything, depending upon its nature, in two ways—instinctively and contemplatively. Let me explain. Suppose you find a snake in your room. Reacting instinctively, you will either run away from the room out of fear or you will fetch a stick to kill the snake. If a snake made of rubber but exactly like a real one is thrown at you, you will first shudder with fear and then realizing that it is made of rubber you may pick it up and admire it and note what a good imitation it is. While your first reaction is instinctive, the subsequent reaction is contemplative. On the other hand, if you see a painting or a sculpture, not imitating but suggesting a snake, you will not react instinctively at all but reacting contemplatively, you will be drawn towards the painting or sculpture with admiration. This reaction is totally contemplative. According to Indian aesthetics, a genuine work of art should not at all arouse an instinctive reaction. The snake made of rubber is *lokadharmi* art, that arouses the instinctive reaction first and later the contemplative. The painting or sculpture suggesting or evoking a snake is *natyadharmi* art that does not arouse the instinctive reaction at all, because it has no *loukika* character and is therefore *aloukika*. According to the *rasa* theory, the showing of different *bhavas* by a dancer or actor, except the humorous and comic, should be *aloukika* to have the character of *natyadharmi*.

Natyadharmi is not abstract, but suggestive and evocative. It has to have a tinge of *loukika* character to be evocative. A mature artist must decide how much of this *loukika* tinge should be given to retain the *natyadharmi* character fully and yet make the presentation highly evocative. Mallarme, a great French poet of the nineteenth century, echoed this aesthetic principle when he said, 'Name a thing and you take away three quarters of its charm. Suggest it, evoke it; that is poetry.' The consideration that a *natyadharmi* presentation should have just a tinge of *loukika* character so that it does not degenerate into *lokadharmi* is termed in the Indian aesthetics as *auchitya*.

The oft-quoted aphorism about the origin of *rasa* in the *Natya Shastra* is:

Vibhava anubhava vyabhichari bhava samjogat rasa nispsth which means that *rasa* issues forth when the *vibhava, anubhava*, and *vyabhichari bhava* are integrated. In order to understand the aphorism one has to correctly understand the deeper implication of these three kinds of *bhavas*.

Vibhava literally means specific *bhava*. As said earlier, *bhava* is the aesthetic evocation of a feeling. As it is, feelings are abstract. If a dancer or actor wants to evoke the feeling of, say, anger, she/he cannot do it without evoking *someone who is angry*. This someone has to be specific, and therefore the *vibhava*. According to the *Natya Shastra*, there are two kinds of *vibhava: alambana vibhava* and *uddipana vibhava*. The former is a specific character, mythological or otherwise, appropriate to evoking a particular kind of feeling. *Alambana* means the receptacle, that is, the character that contains the particular feeling. Therefore, in the field of Indian dance and theatre, the portrayed characters are called *patras*, meaning vessels. *Uddipana* means that which enhances the aesthetic mood. A feeling, at times, requires a particular kind of ambience for enhancing the aesthetic mood. For instance, the evocation of the feeling of love will be enhanced if the dancer suggests through stylized dance movements that it is spring time, many flowers have blossomed and it is a bright moonlit night. This suggestion of an appropriate atmosphere is the *uddipana vibhava*.

Anubhava literally means the *bhava* that follows. Once the *vibhava* is on the stage she/he has to do something to evoke an aesthetic mood. For instance, to give a taste of the aesthetic relish of *karuna* (compassion/pathos) *rasa* the dancer has chosen Rati, the wife of the god of love at the moment after he was burnt to ashes by the angry glare of Lord Shiva, as the *alambana vibhava*. Because of the death of her husband she is stricken with grief (*shoka*). To evoke the feeling of grief she should wear an expression of intense grief on her face, eyes narrowed with sadness and brimming with tears. All these classical expressions and movements are *anubhavas*.

Vyabhichari literally means visitant. Therefore, *vyabhichari bhavas* (also called *sanchari bhava*) are a kind of *anubhavas* which are not naturally associated with a particular kind of feeling, but come in as a visitor in a particular situation. For instance, Radha is always intensely in love with Krishna. When he comes near, her face brightens with love. Then he does not come to her at the appointed time, because he has gone to some other *gopi*. He comes very late to Radha bearing telltale marks of his dalliance with the other *gopi*. Radha is now angry, not radiant, with the nearness of Krishna but this anger is totally different from the regular anger, such as that of Goddess Durga when she comes to fight with Mahishasura. Radha's anger is born out of jealousy (*eersha*) which is a kind of *vyabhichari bhava*.

When all these three kinds of *bhavas* are integrated according to the *auchitya*, the *sthayi bhava* is formed. When the *sthayi bhava* is mentally tasted by the spectator, that particular *rasa* is experienced *sthayi bhava* is ineptly translated as 'Permanent Mental State'. Here the word *sthayi* means resultant rather than permanent. Bharata Muni likens it to *vyanjana* (cooking curry). Like curry, *sthayi bhava* is a preparation with various kinds of ingredients. In a curry, vegetables lose their *loukika* taste and integrated with the spices, acquire an *aloukika* taste. Similarly, in *sthayi bhava*, the various feelings evoked lose their *loukika* character and, integrated with music, costume and dance movements, acquire an *aloukika* character. Like curry, *sthayi bhava* should neither be undercooked nor overcooked. If the *sthayi bhava* retains the *loukika* character of the evoked feelings, then it will be like half-cooked curry, unsuitable for imparting a good taste. Like curry, *sthayi bhava* too has a ruling taste. For instance, the ingredients of a curry, such as some of the spices are bitter, but the ruling taste may be salty, sour or sweet. The *sthayi bhava* may have any of the nine ruling tastes so that the spectator can savour the corresponding *rasa*.

The two words 'artistic' and 'aesthetic' appear to be synonymous, but there is a basic though subtle difference. When a dancer is dancing he/she is engaged in an artistic activity and is having an artistic experience. Those who sit in the audience and watch the performance, have the aesthetic experience. There is nothing like 'aesthetic activity', since it is always an experience. If the artistic activity is of a high order it becomes aesthetically satisfying, i.e. the experience gives a deep satisfaction to the audience.

Just as a part of beautiful eyes cannot see their own beauty, a dancer cannot derive aesthetic satisfaction from her own dancing, since she is at once the artist and the work of art. Other artists are more fortunate. For instance, when a poet is writing a poem he is undergoing the artistic experience. Once the poem is complete, the poet can become its first reader and can have the aesthetic experience. But a pair of eyes requires a mirror to see its own beauty. A dancer similarly requires an audience. If nobody is watching the dancer, the dance is not a performance but a practice (*riaz*). This is why perhaps Indian classical dance traditionally begins after respectfully offering an *anjali* of flowers to the audience.

The much-mouthed but not often rightly understood word *rasa* is basically the aesthetic experience. Just the facial expression of a particular feeling cannot denote a *rasa*. It may be called a *bhava* (which again should never be confused with *sthayi bhava*). The misunderstanding that any expressional/ mimetic passage of the dancing manifests *rasa* has gained so much of currency due to the fact that a few so-called scholars have printed in their highly publicized books, photographs of facial expressions captioned as *rasas*.

The entire seventh chapter of the *Natya Shastra* is devoted to the concept of *bhava* in relation to theatre and dance. This word has *bhu* as its root, literally, coming or bringing into being. If however the causal sense of the word is considered, it means *that which makes one think of something.* Since the meaning of *bhava* is very complex, Indian aestheticians offered a beautiful analogy to deepen the comprehension, of musk (*kasturi*) a highly aromatic substance. If it is rubbed on a kerchief and then put away, the kerchief acquires the aroma of the musk and when it is brought near the nose, it appears as if the musk was 'brought into being' or 'makes one think about the presence of the musk'. The kerchief is thus the *bhava* of *kasturi*. From the perspective of this analogy, *bhava*, so far as dance and theatre are concerned, means a special kind of evocation.

For further elaboration of the subtleties of the Indian *rasa* theory, let us take the example of the *abhinaya* of the well-known *ashtapadi* of Jayadeva, *yahi madhava yahi keshava*, which is danced by almost all the Odissi dancers, but seldom appropriately. On the surface, the words appear to have the charge of anger. If it is so, the lines are then meant to give a taste of *roudra rasa* to the audience. No sensible person will agree to such a preposterous idea, because on examination it will be revealed that the words are more filled with agony than with anger. The Indian aestheticians have clearly indicated that the entire *ashtapadi* is steeped in *shringara rasa* of *vipralamba* kind. The tone of anger comes through the *vyabhichari bhava* named *asooyas* which, according to *Natya Shastra*, is compatible with *shringara rasa*. The treatise has codified the *anubhavas* which can express *asooya*. Even if this subtlety is ignored and it is argued that anger dominates in the words, one has to admit that in a dance presentation the words are not spoken but sung. Does any one in real life sing in anger? If not, how can it be appropriate that the mine structured on sung lines should be lifelike?

In fact, Indian aesthetics does not want any dancer/actor to be a model, but to be a *dhyana padam*. Abhinavagupta in his *Abhinava Bharati* the masterly commentary on the *Natya Shastra*, writes while elaborating on *rasa* :

In a performance the actor/dancer is like a *dhyana padam* for the meditating onlookers. In a temple, an idol worshipped as a deity is actually a *dhyana padam* which literally means a step for meditation. The idol is also called *moorti* which literally means a concretized form. If these two ideas are combined it becomes evident that God who is really formless and infinite is represented by an idol, that is, in a concretized form to serve as the first step for meditation on divinity. Similarly, a dancer while doing *abhinaya*, say for the tasting of *roudra rasa* by the audience, should not try to be a model of an angry man or woman, but the concretized form of anger to serve as the first step for contemplating on the taste of anger. It is very easy to be a model, but a lot of chiselling is required to be transformed into a *dhyana padam*!

Again, from the point of view of disposition, men are divided into three basic categories: *uttama* (noble and dignified), *madyasa* (intermediate), and *adhama* (common or raffish), *abhinaya* of *anubhavas* should accordingly differ. Following this categorization *vaisnava* aestheticians have categorized especially the *nayikas* into *uttama*, *samanjasha* and *sadharani.* The depth and quality of the aspiration to obtain Krishna the Divine, as lover, are the basis of this categorization. That *nayika* belongs to the *sadharani* category who desires Krishna solely for her pleasure without considering whether he will like it or not. Kubja, the hunchback, is placed in this category. A *samanjasham nayika* desires the love of Krishna as much for her pleasure as his. Rukmani for example, comes under this category. There is no trace of selfish motive in the desire of an *uttama nayika* for Krishna. Every atom of her existence is dressed in the pleasure of the Divine. Radha comes under this category. Needless to say that *abhinaya* of the *anubhavas* and *vyabhichari bhavas* has to differ according to the category of the *nayika.*

It is also relevant here to discuss the concept behind the two basic kinds of presentation: *lokadharmi* and *natyadharmi.* According to Indian aesthetics, there are two worlds: *svabhava jagat*, the God-created world which we consider real; and the *vibhava jagat*, the poet-created world which is much larger than life. When the *abhinaya* imitates the *svabhava jagat*, it is called *lokadharmi*, that is realistic, but when it evokes the *vibhava jagat* it is *natyadharmi*. The latter being suggestive and evocative is considered more artistic.

No doubt, dance is an applied *prayogatamaka* art. The dancer therefore needs to know how to and what to apply. Mastering the techniques of a particular art/dance style gives the dancer the right answer to the question, how to apply. But it is the thorough understanding of the *rasa* theory that can give him/her the right answer to question what to apply. If one does not know the latter the former becomes empty and sterile. India, down the centuries, has held that in the field of art *rasameva jayate*, which means 'it is only *rasa* that is celebrated'.

The Six Limbs of Dance

According to the traditional Indian thinking the way a dancer combines the movements of all her limbs is essentially not different from the way a painter arranges forms and colours in his painting. Both are artists and through their art they seek to explore some of the countless facets of beauty which may for some time taxi in the plane of forms and colours but finally does take off to the plane of the formless and colourless. If it does not take off, it is only an imitation, not the genuine thing. To Indian thinkers, the dichotomy between concrete and abstract is irrelevant since it is the formless that manifests itself in forms, and the colourless in colours. Viewed from this perspective, dance and painting are but two facets of the same thing and the principles of one are well applicable to the other.

In a sense, art like its creators, the artists, is a being. If a human being has six limbs (two legs, the torso, two hands and the head), any art, be it painting or dancing or any other form of art, has six limbs. The *Kamasutra* and many other Sanskrit texts discuss the *sadanga*, i.e. six limbs of the art of painting. The *Abhinayachandrika*, though a treatise on Odissi dance, has many things that are applicable to any other form of classical dance. It says that without the knowledge of *sadanga* the dance falls to the level of folk dancing (*vinoo sadanga jnaanena nritya deshi sajayate*). Obviously, the *sadanga* here does not refer to the limbs like legs or hands but to the six limbs of the art of painting.

Sadanga, the six principles of Indian painting are: (i) *Roopa-bheda*, (ii) *Sadrishya*, (iii) *Bhava*, (iv) *Lavanya yojana*, (v) *Pramana*, and (vi) *Varnikabhanga*. If likened to the limbs of a human being, they may respectively be the two hands, the two legs and the torso.

(i) *Roopa-bheda*: Literally, it means 'the distinction of forms'. The painter or the dancer must know that there are many forms which although similar in appearance, are distinctly different. For instance, a lotus and a water lily have many similarities so far as form is concerned, but are different flowers. Therefore, an accomplished dancer, like a painter, knows how to delineate each in the danced dimension. The subtler implication of the principle of *roopa-bheda* comes into consideration when a dancer, say, is delineating rain. The delineation should clearly suggest whether it is drizzling or pouring, in keeping with the *sthayi bhava* of the situation.

(ii) *Sadrishya*: Literally it means 'resemblance', but it implies that the artists must know the symbolic and/or spiritual significance of the forms and appearances they visually present. Again, this principle claims careful consideration when a dancer is dealing with a metaphorical passage. For example, if the expression 'lotus eyed' is being delineated in a dance, the dancer has to know why the eye has *sadrishya* with the lotus and not with, say, a water lily or rose or *champak*.

(iii) *Bhava*: It means 'aesthetic feelings' and perhaps needs no explanation so far dance is concerned.

(iv) *Lavanya yojana*: It means 'planning for gracefulness'. A painter fills the area of the two-dimensional canvas with various forms and colours. Even if he uses quite pleasing colours on graceful forms, without any planning, the painting as a whole will appear unbalanced and therefore aesthetically irritating rather than pleasing. Similarly, a dancer fills the three-dimensional stage space with dance movements. Even if she is very pretty, wears a beautiful costume, and her movements are as graceful as they are sensuous, if the presentation has no planning, which means it has not been choreographed well, it may irritate sensitive spectators.

(v) *Pramana*: It means 'proportions of arrangements' and is essentially linked with *lavanya yojana*. Sweetness is no doubt a pleasant sensation of the tongue, but too much sweetness is unpleasant. An accomplished dancer knows that too many graceful movements may impart a sloppy character to her performance.

(vi) *Varnikabhanga*: It generally means 'harmonization of colours'. This perhaps needs no explanation in the art of painting. In dance, however, its subtler implication is to be taken into consideration. Even if the literal meaning of the term is taken into consideration, it points to the *aharya* (costume and makeup) of the dancer. Dancing is but an aesthetic pattern for the sensitive eyes and ears of a spectator. A dancer should know that when the accompanying music appeals to the ear, her movements as much as *aharya* appeals to the eye. Therefore, if the costume she wears has incongruous and unharmonized colours, it will irritate the eyes of a sensitive spectator. As a result, her performance will lose some of its appeal if the *aharya* does not follow the principles of *varnikabhanga*.

The System and Tradition of Odissi Music

IF ANY REGIONAL style of music of this country claims a distinctive and shastric system, then it has to satisfy the following points:

(a) The tradition is more than one century old.
(b) The system is based on one or more written *shastras*.
(c) There are a number of *ragas* at the core of the system even if the number is less than one hundred, and
(d) The *ragas* at the core of the system and those borrowed from other systems are delineated in a distinctive style.

If any of the above points is not satisfied then it may get the acceptance of a distinctive style, but cannot get the acceptance as a separate and distinctive system. Let us now see if Odissi music (which perhaps in ancient times was called Odra *Sangeet*) can satisfy the above points.

Tradition

About half a century ago, the renowned scholar and researcher Mahamahopadhyaya Haraprasad Shastri discovered in Nepal some *charya* songs which are meant to be sung in the rituals connected with Buddhist Tantrism. A detailed study of these *charya* songs reveals that they were written between the ninth and eleventh centuries and the poets came mainly from Orissa and Bengal. These fifty *charya* songs have been published as a book called *Budha Gaan O Doha*. Very similar to the Chhanda tradition of Orissa, each of these songs is meant to be sung in a particular *raga*. The language used in the songs is an interesting mixture of Oriya, Bengali and Assamese. Therefore, it can be assumed that almost a thousand years ago, eastern India had one language from which these three languages emerged later.

The fifty *charya* songs which Dr. Shastri discovered were set in the following *ragas*:

1. Twelve songs in *Patamanjari raga*;
2. Five in *Mallari*;
3. Four each in *Baradi*, *Kamod* and *Bhairavi*;
4. Three each in *Gujari* and *Gabura*;
5. Two each in *Deshakhya*, *Ramakeri* and *Shavari*;
6. One each in *Devakiri*, *Dhanyasi*, *Malasi*, *Bengal*, *Kanhugunjari*, etc.

These were composed by twenty-three Buddhist Tantric poets. It is a fact that Orissa had been one of the main centres of both Buddhism and Tantrism. Again, out of the eighteen *ragas* in which the *charya* songs were set except for *Gabura*, *Aru* and *Indralata*, the definition of the other fifteen *ragas* is found in *Geeta Prakash* and *Sangeet Narayana* which were

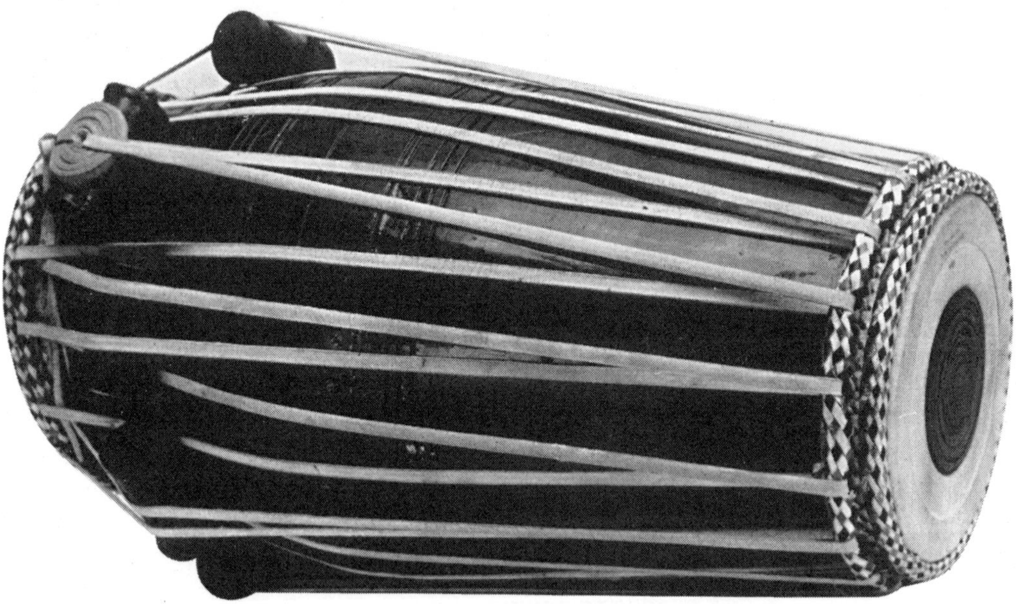

6. *Mardal*—a dancer's life. Photo: SNA, New Delhi.

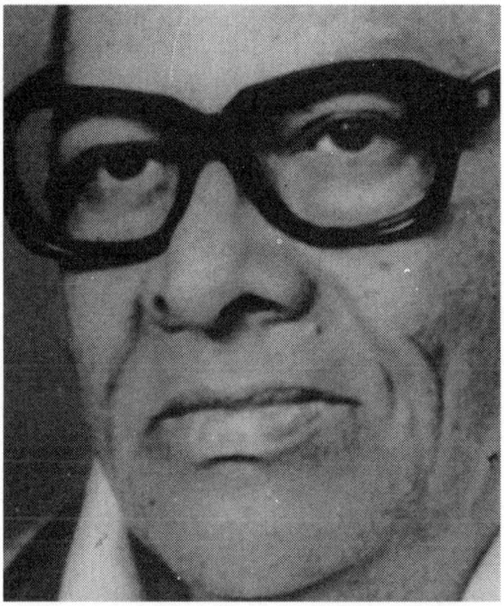

7. Sangeet Sudhakar Balakrishna Dash

written in Orissa. Most probably, *Indralata* is the name of a *tala*, not a *raga*. Mention of *Gabura* and *Aru* is not found in any music treatise of India. Most probably, these two *ragas* gradually got consumed in other *ragas* or because they had strong folk elements, they could not be accepted as *shastric ragas*. This will be more clear if the *Shavari raga* is studied in its historical perspective.

The twenty-sixth and thirty-sixth *charya* songs are required to be sung in *Shavari*. From its name and also from its *dhyanashloka*, it is clear that the *raga* is the product of the culture of a non-Aryan community called Shavara. It is culture that has given Orissa the well-known Jagannatha cult. The twenty-eighth *charya* song has been composed by one 'Shavara', although it is set to *Raga Varati*. This word 'Shavara' perhaps indicates the community rather than the name of the poet. Whatever it may be, it seems a safe assumption, that the *Raga Shavari* has come from the Shavara culture.

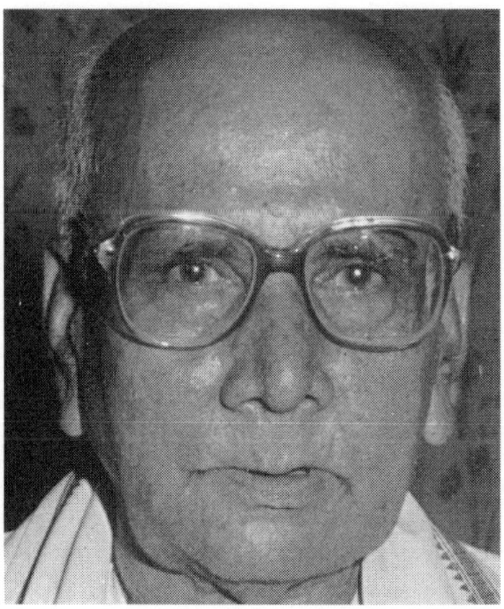

8. Kasinath Pujapanda

The earliest mention of the *Raga Shavari* is found in the *Sangeeta Ratnakara* of Sarangadeva (thirteenth century AD). In this monumental treatise on music, *Shavari* has been spelt as *Savari*. This negligible difference may be owing to the mistake of the scribes or because in Oriya the three sibilants in the alphabet are pronounced only as the dental sibilant. In the *Sangeeta Ratnakara*, *Shavari* has been included under the category of 'now well-known *Bhasanga ragas*'. Therefore, it may be assumed that by the thirteenth century, the *raga* had found its place in all Indian *shastric* music. But during the eighth century, it was not accepted as a *raga*, which is evident from the following quotation from Matanga's *Brihaddeshi*:

चतुः स्वरात् प्रवृति न मार्गः।
शवर-पुलिन्द-काम्बोज-वंग-किरात-
अन्ध्र-द्राविर-वनादिषु प्रयुज्जते।

From this quotation it may be assumed that in the eighth century, most probably, *Shavari* was being sung with four notes. Moreover, not only *Shavari* but *Pulindi*, *Kamboji*, *Bangala*, *Andhri ragas* which later were accepted as part of *shastric* music, were also sung with four notes at least until the eighth century.

During the period between the ninth and eleventh centuries (when the *charya* songs were composed), it seems that *Raga Shavari* had got a place in the *prabandha gayana* style because the 292nd *shloka* of the chapter on the *prabandha gayana* in the *Sangeeta Ratnakara* says:

पद्धड़ी प्रभृति छन्दाः पादान्त प्रासशोभिता
अध्यात्मगोचरो चर्या स्याद् द्वितीयादि तालतः।

As a commentary to this couplet, Kallinatha has said:

पदतालबद्धत्वात् द्वयंग।
तारा वली जातिमान्।

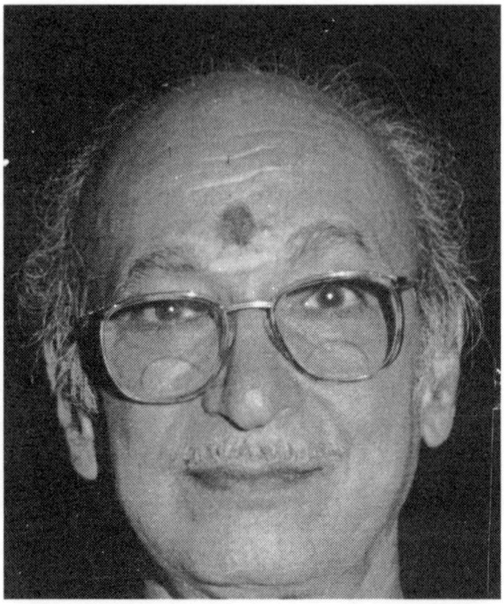

9. Sangeet Suramani Raghunath Panigrahi

From these two quotations it is clear that at least by the time of the thirteenth century, the style of singing *charya* songs were accepted under the *taravali* kind of *prabandhas*. The ancient shape of Odissi music was of this kind of *prabandha* singing. Thus, the tradition of Odissi music is at least one thousand years old.

Shastra

If a dance or music style does not follow *shastras* then it cannot be called *shastric*. If Indian culture is deeply studied, it will be revealed that any regional culture has two aspects:

(a) Pan-Indian elements
(b) Distinct regional elements.

Probably because of this, despite the amazing variety, Indian culture has remained unified for centuries. Odissi dance has been accepted as a *shastric* tradition because it follows two kinds of *shastras*, one pan-Indian (*Natya Shastra* and *Abhinaya Darpana*) and the other, regional, *Abhinayachandrika* and other dance treatises written in Orissa.

Odissi music similarly follows the *Natya Shastra* and the *Sangeeta Ratnakara* of Sarangadeva for its pan-Indian aspects and *Geeta Prakashan* and *Sangeet Narayana*, which were written between the sixteenth and eighteenth century in Orissa, for its regional distinctiveness. At present, the following treatises of Odissi music are available in the form of published books:

1. *Geeta Prakash* by Krishnadas Badajena Mahapatra—AD 1565
2. *Sangeeta Kalpalatika* by Hardhar Mishra—between AD 1619 and 1644
3. *Natyamanorama* by Raghunath Rath—AD 1696
4. *Sangeet Narayana* by Gajapati Narayan Dev—AD 1750
5. *Sangeet Muktavali* by Hari Chandan (after AD 1750)

Of the above mentioned treatises, the most important are *Geeta Prakash* and *Sangeet Narayana*, since they contain definitions of the *ragas* that formed the core of the system.

A deep study of the *shastras* will reveal that although they follow the *Sangeeta Ratnakara*, they differ at times, which proves the regional distinctiveness of the system.

For instance, let us consider the *Raga Vasanta*. According to the *Sangeeta Ratnakara* (vide *Raga Vivekadhayaya*, Chapter 2, *shlokas* 93-6), the *raga* is born from the pentatonic *Hindola raga*. If *Hindola* is made haptatonic, it becomes *Vasanta* which comes under both *Dhaivati* and *Arshabhi jati* (ancient scales, prior to *ragas*). But in Odra *Sangeet* (the ancient music of Orissa), *Vasanta* is a totally different *raga*.

Both *Geeta Prakash* and *Sangeet Narayana* mention that *Vasanta* is born of the *Susdjamadhyamika jati* which is under *Matsarikrita Moorchana*, if the notes used in the *Moorchana* are converted to the notes used in the Hindustani music system, then the *Moorchana* will be more or less like the *Khamaj Thaat*. This proves that Odissi music, although it followed the *Natya Shastra* and *Sangeeta Ratnakara*, maintained its distinctive identity, at least in respect of some *ragas*.

Moreover, *ragas* such as *Hunchhika*, *Bhauli*, *Tara*, *Salagagouda*, *Megharanji*, etc., are not mentioned in the *Sangeeta Ratnakara*. Thus, it is proved that the musical tradition prevalent in Orissa had a distinctive system of its own based on the *shastras* written in this particular region.

Core Ragas

Be it Karnataka or Hindustani systems of music, each has a number of *ragas* at its core. These *ragas* are more important than the *ragas* borrowed from other systems. The *ragas* which have been mentioned by the said *shastras* form the core *ragas* of the Odissi system of music. At present, *ragas* such as *Kafi*, *Mohana*, *Keervani* are very popular but they are all borrowed. Therefore, they should have been less important than the core *ragas*. It is indeed very unfortunate that the present day Odissi musicians have almost forgotten the core *ragas* of the Odra system and give more importance to borrowed *ragas*. Only *Shankarabharana*, *Shavari* (which is being wrongly spelt as *Savari*), *Bhairavi* and *Mukhabari* (*Mukhari*) are the few core *ragas* which are still being sung although not using notes as indicated by the Odissi *shastras* which mention more than 75 *ragas*. As a result, this rich tradition of music is getting distorted day by day.

Rendition Style

The most important characteristic of any system of music, is its distinctive style of *raga* delineation. For example, the *Hindolam raga* of the Karnataka system and the *Malkauns* of Hindustani use the same notes but the rendition of the *raga* is different since different *gamakas* are used in each style. The Odra system of music uses yet another kind of *gamaka* for *raga* delineation. The Odissi style of music has again two branches of the rendition style:

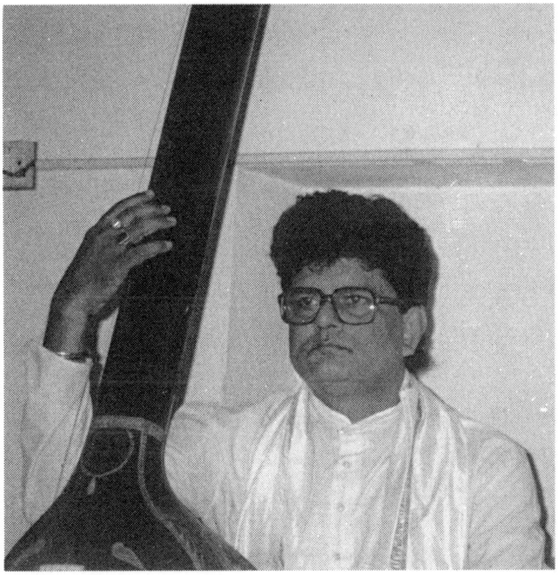

10. Bankim Sethi

(a) *geeta* singing and
(b) *chhanda* singing

Of these two, *chhanda* singing is simpler and has some non-shastric elements but the style of singing of *geetas* is highly evolved. The difference between the *khayal* singing of Hindustani system and the rendition of *geetas* in Odissi sysem is that while the former lays more emphasis on the correct use of notes, the latter emphasizes on the emotional content of the song. In this respect, the Odra style is somewhat similar to the Karnataka system.

From the discussions above, it is evident that Odissi music is a distinctive *shastric* system. Again, it is now accepted that Odissi dance is undoubtedly a *shastric* style. Undoubtedly, music is the life breath of dance. Therefore, it will not be logical to say that the body, that is the Odissi dance, is *shastric*, but its life, i.e. the music, is not *shastric*. Even the query about why Odissi music is not being accepted as a distinctive *shastric* system deserves to be discussed. Firstly, the way Odissi songs are now being rendered is not totally traditional. It is true that the tradition is like a flow and therefore it is natural that it will undergo certain changes, but the changed form should not be so different as to have no relation to the source.

There are a number of knowledgeable Odissi musicians who can give an adequate idea about the distinctive style of Odissi music. The author had the opportunity of discussing

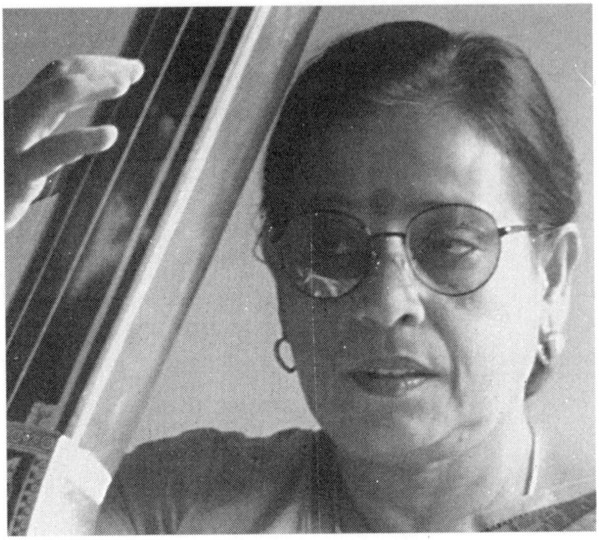

11. Bhubaneswari Mishra

the matter with the well-known vocalist Smt. Veenapani Mishra. She clearly demonstrated the distincitve gamakas which are used in Odissi music. I am sure, such knowledgeable musicians like Markandeya Mahapatra, Balakrishna Dash, Bhubaneswari Mishra, Damodar Hota, Gopal Chandra Panda and young musicians and researchers like Ramahari Das and Bankim Sethi can throw a good deal of light on the distinctive style of rendition of the Odissi *ragas*. It is indeed unfortunate that Orissa has such talented musicians and such knowledgeable scholars such as Neela Madhava Panigrahi, yet Odissi music is going around with a begging bowl and even going to the extent of borrowing certain cheap and glamorous elements from film music. One has to be a stubborn optimist to hope that the day will come when the said talented musicians and knowledgeable scholars will combine to give Odissi music the *shastric* stature which it had even less than a hundred years ago.

Krishna in Odissi Dance

THE KRISHNA-RADHA legend fascinated poets and playwrights of Orissa, writing in Sanskrit, from around the seventh century when Bhatta Narayana authored the play titled *Venisamaharam*. Although the play is based on the story of Draupadi's humiliation, which was avenged by Bhima, the second *Mangalacharana* eulogizes Krishna and Radha. It says, 'When in a fit of sulks Radha left the *rasa* dance, to mollify her Krishna was following by stepping on her footsteps, he was getting gooseflesh.' There are many such lines in other works of literature, but Odissi dance was inundated with the Krishna-Radha legend from the twelfth century onwards influenced by the *Geetagovinda* of Jayadeva.

The sculptural evidence of the first century BC at Ranigumpa and several treatises on Odissi dance (earlier known as Odra *nritya*) written between the sixteenth and nineteenth centuries point to the fact that three classes of dancers were performing this style of dance. The *nartakis* were dancing in the royal courts and for the general public in the traditional festivals like Vasantotsava. The aim of their dance was to give aesthetic relish (*rasanubhuti*) to the audience. The *maharis* and *devadasis* used to perform in the temples and their dance was basically ritualistic. From around the seventeenth century, another class of dancers called *gotipua* began to perform the dance for the mass. Their dance was aesthetically satisfying, but with a touch of popular appeal. Owing to extreme changes in social values and gradual withdrawal of royal patronage, the *nartakis* were the first to disappear from the scene by around the latter half of the nineteenth century. The *maharis* continued to dance in the temple of Lord Jagannatha at Puri till the fourth decade of this century, but their dance had so much decayed that it was more a ritual than dance.

The expressional numbers of the *nartakis* till the twelfth century were mostly based on Sanskrit poems, often steeped in *Shringara-rasa*, but not inspired by the Krishna legend. But the *Geetagovinda* became so popular that both the *nartakis* and *maharis* began basing their expressional numbers freqently on its *ashtapadis*.

Singing and dancing of *ashtapadis* became the regular form of temple service from around the thirteenth century. It was disrupted for some time, but Prataparudra Dev, the Gajapati king of Puri, restarted it. On 8 July 1500, he proclaimed that no song and dance other than those based on the *Geetagovinda* should be performed inside the temple of Lord Jagannatha. The proclamation was also inscribed on the Jayavijaya gate inside the temple.

In fact, Jayadeva shaped the *Geetagovinda* as a *sangeetaka*, an *uparoopaka*, that is, a play with music and dance. His wife Padmavati was a *mahari* and performed expressional numbers based on his *ashtapadis* within the Jagannatha temple. The *gotipuas* were performing expressional numbers mostly on Oriya poems written between seventeenth and nineteenth century. They also, at times, used to perform *ashtapadis*. The influence of the *Geetagovinda* was so deep that the highly ornate Oriya poetry of the said period was immensely inspired by the Krishna legend.

In the twelfth century, four great Vaishnava saints from south India came to Puri and established their respective *maths* (monasteries). They are Vishnu Swami, Ramanujancharya, Acharya Nimbarka and Madhvacharya. Scholars are of the opinion that Jayadeva was influenced by the Vaishnavism professed by Acharya Nimbarka. All four spiritual leaders identified Lord Jagannatha with Krishna. The pre-Chaitanya Vaishnavism in Orissa was *jnana-mishra-bhakti* (devotion steeped in metaphysical knowledge) whereas Chaitanyadev professed *shuddhaprema-bhakti* (devotion steeped in pure love) which is known as Goudiya Vaishnavism. In the sixteenth century Chaitanyadev came to Puri. Although he accepted that Krishna and Jagannatha are one and the same, some of his Bengali disciples did not accept it and being angry they came back to Nadia in Bengal. Chaitanyadev remained in Puri till he breathed his last.

Krishna and Radha originally belonged to the pantheon of the Abhirs, a highly cultured non-Aryan pastoral community. When the Abhir culture merged into Aryan culture, Krishna was accepted as a god of the latter's pantheon and was identified with Vishnu, but Radha had to wait for centuries to be regarded as an Aryan goddess. There are, of course, several references to the dancing of Krishna, Radha and the *gopis* in the literary works of great poets like Kalidasa. In the twelfth century, Acharya Nimbarka initiated the worship of Radha and Krishna together. It is he who in his *Dashashloki* described Radha as a goddess. The following *shloka* from the said devotional poem perhaps is the first that regarded Radha not only as the beloved of Krishna but also as a goddess:

'The daughter of Vrishabhanu (i.e. Radha) like Lakshmi remains happily on the left side (of Krishna). A thousand

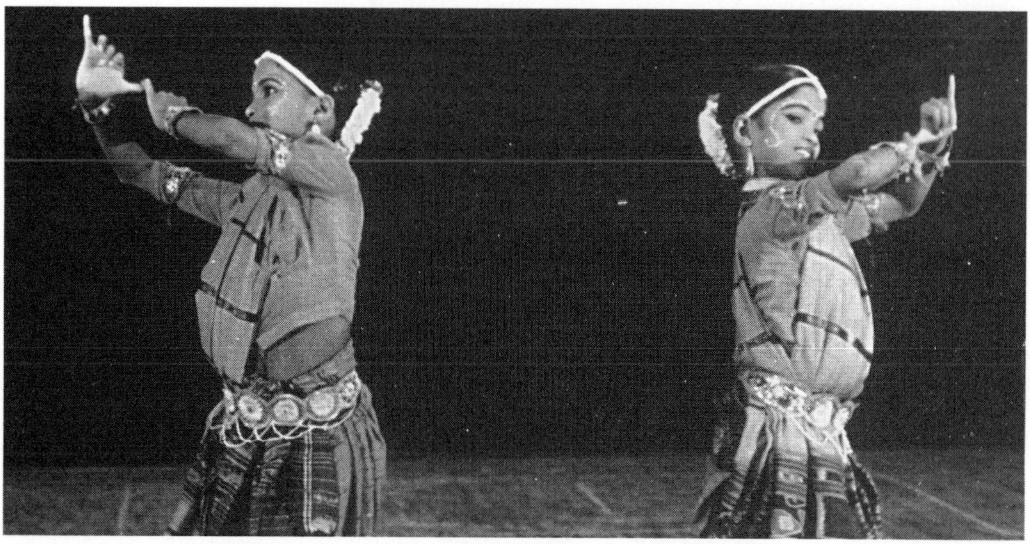

12. *Gotipuas* in dancing postures. Photo: SNA, New Delhi.

maidens surrounding her serve her. Always, I reverentially remember the goddess who fulfils all that is blissful and all that one desires.'

Gradually various orders of Vaishnavism as also the Aryan culture accepted Radha as a goddess. Till the twelfth century both Krishna and Radha were mythological characters, but in Vaishnavism the duo became concepts rather than mythical characters. In Orissa, Krishna was more popular as Madhava, one of his myriad synonyms. He was worshipped in many different temples identified with Vishnu. After the *Geetagovinda* the worship of Radha-Madhava became popular. Jayadeva has eulogized Radha-Madhava in the *mangalacharan* of the *Geetagovinda*, the concluding line of which reads:

'Glory to Radha-Madhava, who on the bank of the river Yamuna secretly had love play.'

According to Chaitanyadev and many other great Vaishnava saints, the *Geetagovinda* is a *dharma grantha* (religious scripture). Chaitanyadev went to the extent of proclaiming that the *Geetagovinda* is the best prayer to Krishna ever written. The Vaishnavas do not consider it as merely erotic because they understand the subtle metaphysical symbolism inherent in the poem. If the allegorical symbolism inherent in poems inspired by the Krishna legend is ignored, they will appear highly erotic, bordering on pornography. If the Odissi dancers who perform expressional numbers based on such poems do not adequately understand the symbolism, their *abhinaya* will be shallow, I will therefore very briefly discuss the allegorical symbolism.

As said earlier, Krishna and Radha in Vaishnavism after the twelfth century are concepts rather than mythological characters. Their relationship is likened to the sugar (*madhu*) and sweetness (*madhurata*). They are eternally united and cannot be separated. We intellectually separate sweetness from sugar. Similarly, Radha is separated from Krishna only for the *leela*. Therefore, in Vaishnava philosophy, Krishna-

Radha appear in two forms: *nitya roopa*, the eternal form in which they are ever united and are inseparable, and the *leela roopa*, the temporal form in which they are separated. Jayadeva has put it across very subtly in the seventh *ashtapadi* that describes how Krishna is searching for the sulking Radha. In the sixth shloka he says to himself:

'If I eternally hold her in a tight embrace in my heart and constantly caress her, why am I unnecessarily searching her in this forest and why do I feel so dejected?'

After saying this he still searches for her. Jayadeva has subtly hinted that Krishna had a flash of his *nitya roopa* while in his *leela roopa*. Right from the time of the *Bhagavata Purana*, which mentions, not Radha, but only the *gopis*, Krishna has been conceived as a divinity beyond time and space, and having no physical presence in the real sense of the term. The episode of *vastra-haran* in which Krishna takes away the clothes of the *gopis* while they were bathing is crucial. He symbolically indicates to his devotees that he has no physical presence and therefore there is no reason for the *gopis* to be ashamed before him, especially since they consider him as *antaryami*, which literally means 'who goes inside'. Krishna, therefore, can only be experienced, not perceived by the five senses. And Vaishnavas consider Radha as the *hladini shakti*, meaning the ecstasy-giving energy. The love between them is beyond body and beyond time and space. An eighteenth century Oriya poet, Abhimanya Samanta Singhaar, has beautifully expressed it in his *kavya*: *Vidagdha Chintamani*, which is quoted below:

लाख घोड़ा नवनीत सुआर
प्रचण्डानलें पथ चालिबार
तहुँ कि करि रहिब शरीर
तहुँ अधिक प्रीति पालिबार।।

It means 'A horse made of sealing wax, on it the rider is made of butter. Both are running on a road that is all a flame. How can their body remain as they are? (The two bodies will melt and mingle and finally go up in smoke.) Love is beyond that state.'

This wonderful imagery indicates the mystique of the love between Krishna and Radha. There are countless such lines in the vast body of Oriya poetry, inspired by the Krishna legend.

The Odissi dance (earlier known as Odra *nritya*) has thus been very deeply influenced by Vaishnavism from the twelfth century onwards. Therefore, it will be a travesty if an Odissi dancer ignores the symbolism while performing expressional numbers based on poems inspired by the Krishna legend. I have grave doubts that the *gurus* who are now imparting training in Odissi dance have any idea of the deep and poetic symbolism behind the Krishna legend. Therefore, when they compose expressional numbers based on the Krishna legend they depict him as an ordinary human lover, philandering with countless girls. In such compositions, Krishna, the divine lover beyond time and space and having no physical presence, appears as a super Casanova. How does this reconcile with the allegorical wealth of Odissi?

The Tradition of Mahari Dance

ODRA *NRITYA* (NOW popularly known as Odissi) evolved out of the ritual dancing of the consecrated girls called *devadasis.* These ritual dancers attached to the temple of Lord Jagannatha at Puri, are known as *maharis.* They performed inside the temple every day at specified times and their dance was regarded as one of the thirty-six essential temple services (*niyoga*). The tradition started declining from the eighteenth century and survived till the third decade of twentieth century, almost worn to a shadow, it is now more than forty years since a *mahari* has danced inside the temple premises.

In fact, there were two kinds of *maharis*, the singing (*gauni*) *mahari* and the dancing (*nachuni*) *mahari.* Although the *mahari* dance is extinct, the tradition of singing lines from Jayadeva's *Geetagovinda* by a *gauni mahari* still survives though in an emaciated form. The only surviving authentic *gauni mahari* is Kokilapriya who is now around sixty.

A frew treatises on Odissi music and dance written between the fifteenth and the eighteenth century are still extant. Of these *Abhinayachandrika* by Maheshwara Mahapatra (fifteenth century) deals most elaborately with the dance tradition. It does not, however, mention the *maharis* or *devadasis* and the manner in which it describes the qualities of a dancer and a few dance postures, unmistakably points to the fact that, at the time when it was written, there were two kinds of Odissi dancers: the *devadasi* in the temple, and

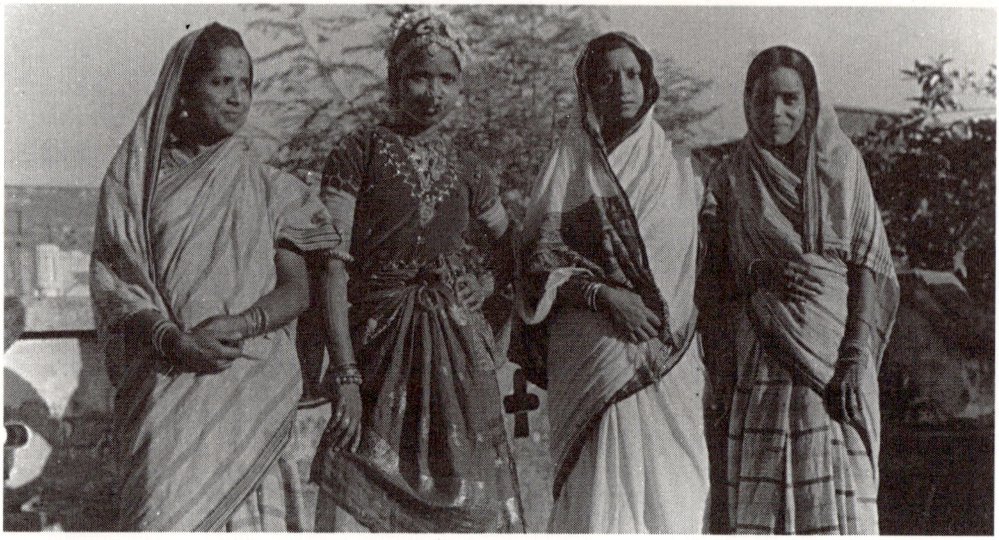

13. The traditional *maharis* of Puri. Photo: SNA, New Delhi.

the *nachuni* in the royal court. Most probably Maheshwara Mahapatra was a *guru* of the court dancers.

Before any reason is offered as to why the word *mahari* finds no mention in an elaborate treatise like the *Abhinaya-chandṛika*, it is necessary to explain what exactly the word means. So far no satisfactory etymological meaning of *mahari* has been forthcoming. One point of view states, 'the *nari* (woman) who is *mahat* (auspicious) is *mahari*'. This explanation is not tenable. According to the rules of Sanskrit grammar, *mahat-nari* becomes *mahannari*, which in colloquial language may become *mannari*, but it is almost impossible that it should become *mahari*. The *Bhagavata Puran* says that, at the time of *pralaya* (universal deluge), genuine devotees of Vishnu took shelter in *maharaloka*, the celestial world or extra-terrestrial area of existence (heaven). In fact, the concept of seven *lokas* in Indian philosophy and mythology is unique. The word '*loka*' is derived from the root '*lok*' meaning 'to see' or 'to perceive' or 'to experience'. Therefore, *loka* is a level of experience and the *saptalokas* in ascending order are *bhu*, *bhova*, *svarga*, *mahara*, *jana*, *tapa* and *satya*. The highest *loka*, i.e. *Satyaloka*, is also called *Brahmaloka*. According to Vaishnavism, there are nine *lokas*. Above *Satya-loka* is *Vaikuntha*, and the highest is *Goloka* where Lord

Krishna resides perpetually. The word '*go*' does not (as is generally believed) mean 'a cow' alone; it primarily means 'ray' or 'light'. Many words compounded with '*go*' would make no sense if the meaning is interpreted as 'cow'. For instance, gomati, which is the name of a river, etymologically means 'she who possesses *go*'. Here, if the meaning of *go* is interpreted as 'cow', the connotation of the compound word (*gomati*) becomes quite strange—a river in which cows swim like fish. The other meaning, however, makes sense, a river that shines. Thus, *Goloka* is the level where not cows but pure light is experienced.

In Hindu mythology there are countless references to dancing in the *Svargaloka.* The dancers there are called *apsaras* which, literally means 'those women who have moved up from the surface of water'. What a poetic conception! The dancer who dances in *Svargaloka* does not have a body like that of a human being, on which gravitational force perpetually works, but a beautiful etheral body made up of clouds of various hues which rise from the surface of the sea. The aim of an *apsara's* dance is to give the audience aesthetic entertainment of the highest order. The aim of a *devadasi's* dance goes much beyond, since it is a prayer, a form of worship. When a dancer, while performing, reaches the highest aesthetic level she experiences *Svargaloka*, but if she goes still higher, she reaches *Maharaloka.* In conformity with the rules of Sanskrit grammar, the people of *mahara* are called *mahara*, the feminine gender of which is *mahari.* This, in spoken Oriya, became *mahari.*

Originally, the institution of *devadasi* was undoubtedly Tantrik. The Jagannatha cult is a unique synthesis of several, often divergent, religious precepts. From the twelfth century, when Jayadeva wrote the famous *Geetagovinda* the Vaishnava aspect of the cult began to predominate, but even today, elements of Tantrik ritual are very much in evidence in the worship of Lord Jagannatha. The much misunderstood *pancha-makara puja* of Tantra is followed somewhat in Jagannatha worship. The five *makaras* are *madya* (wine), *matsya* (fish), *mamsa* (meat), *mudra* (money) and *maithuna* (sex). In the worship of Jagannatha they are also hypostatized in the following manner:

(i) water of a green coconut kept in a vessel made of bell metal represents *madya* (wine); (ii) vegetables cooked with asafoetida represent *matsya* (fish); (iii) thinly chopped ginger represents *mamsa* (meat); (iv) a variety of roasted beans represent *mudra* (money) and (v) the dance of a *devadasi* represents *maithuna* (sex).

There are a few inscriptions to prove that the tradition of *devadas* dancing in the temples of Orissa was prevalent before the eleventh century. It may be surmised that *devadas* attached to the Jagannatha temple at Puri were named *mahari* after the fifteenth century, since the inscription on the Jayavijaya *dvara* of the temple (dated AD 8 July 1500), refers to four different groups of *devadasis* employed under the temple service. They are (i) *Purana sampradaya* (the ancient group); (ii) *Badathakuranka sampradaya* (the group attached to Balabhadra), (iii) *Kapileshwara sampradaya* (the group belonging to Kapileshwara), and (iv) *Tailangi sampradaya* (the group of the Telengana region).

In this inscription, the consecrated dancers are neither referred to as *devadasi* nor as *mahari*, but, as *bandha nachuni* which literally means 'bonded dancer' and connotes 'formally and permanently engaged dancer'. In the sixteenth century, during the rule of Prataparudra Deva, who was a devout Vaishnava, the Jagannatha cult came to be considerably influenced by Vaishnavism. It may be surmised that from this period the *devadasis* of the temple were known as *maharis*. This also explains why the term *mahari* was not used in *Abhinayachandrika* in the fifteenth century.

Although the treatise does not mention either *mahari* or *devadasi*, it refers on several occasions to and describes *batu-nritya* which, if properly analysed, will undoubtedly point to the dance of the *maharis*. Before the references are analysed let us examine what exactly *batu-nritya* means.

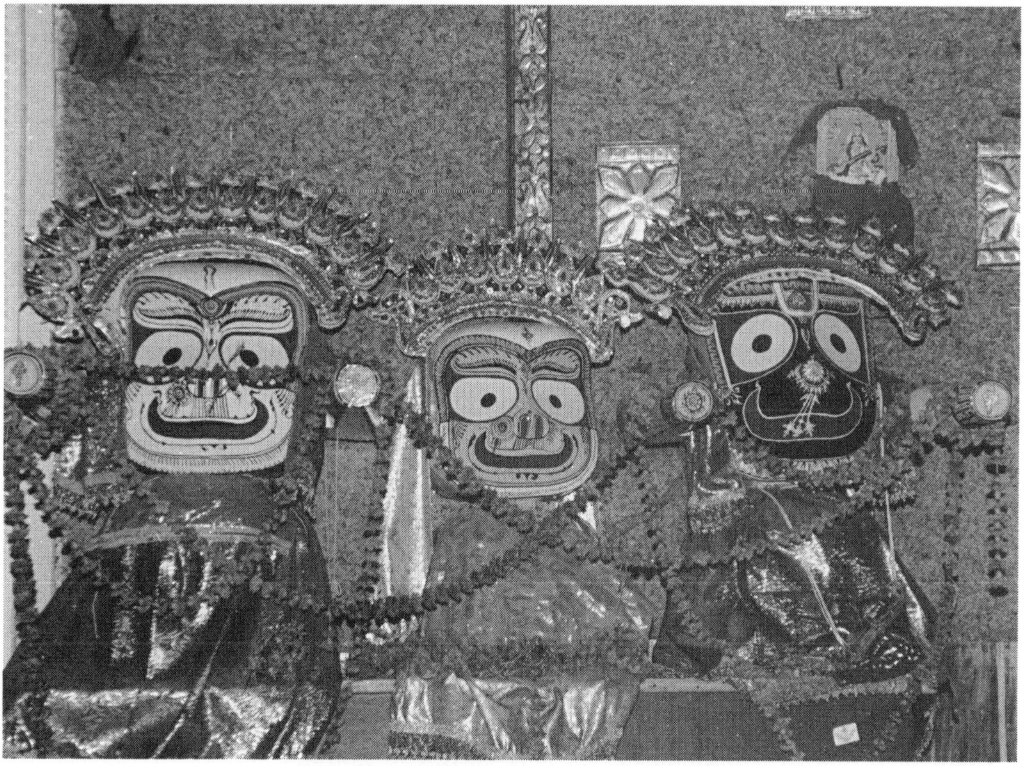

14. The three deities, Balabhadra, Subhadra and Jagannatha. Photo: Dillip Tripathy.

In eastern India, especially in Orissa and Bengal, the Sanskrit letter *va* is pronounced as *ba*. Therefore, the Sanskrit, word '*vatu*' becomes *batu* in Oriya. *Vatu* is derived from the root *vat* which, in Sanskrit, is defined in two ways. Under the first (*bhavadi*) class of verbs and the tenth (*churadi*) class of verbs, it generally means 'to surround' or 'to be'. In the former sense, *vatu* is compounded with *kusha* (a kind of grass) to form *kushavatu* which is a ring made of *kusha* grass worn on the ring finger during the performance of some religious rites. In the latter sense (i.e. to be) *vatu* generally means a Brahmin male of adolescent age (spanning the period from his sacred thread ceremony to his marriage). This is because during this period he is 'tied' to the *brahmacharya vrata* (the vow of celibacy). The most elaborate and authentic Oriya lexicon is *Purnachandra Oriya Bhashakosha.* On page 5307 of the lexicon, under the word '*batu*', the compiler

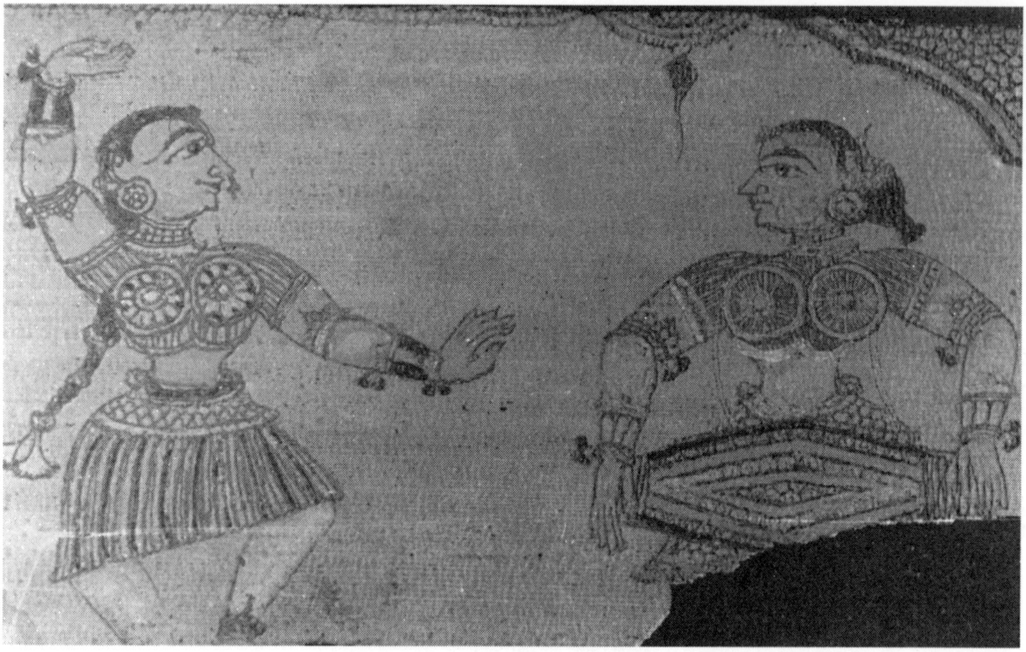

15. A dancer dancing before a musician. *Gitagovinda* palmleaf manuscript, National Archieves, New Delhi Collections.

has indicated that in colloquial Oriya, it is known as *badu.* And on page 5315 of the same work, under *badu* are listed the following three meanings:

(1) The *brahamachari* after the sacred thread ceremony;
(2) A gardener engaged in the temple service of Lord Lingaraj at Bhubaneswar;
(3) An attendant, a servant.

In fact, a servant who is bound to do a particular kind of work daily or at regular intevals is called *badu.* Many *sevakas* (temple servants), attached to the Jagannatha temple at Puri, who do a particular kind of *seva* (temple service), have been designated by compounding *badu* with the kind of service that each is bound to do regularly during the various rituals to worship Lord Jagannatha. They are designated as *patri badu*, *suara badu*, *vimana badu*, *khatua badu*, *tola badu*, *gara badu* and so on. In the Sanskritized version, *badu* becomes *batu*. For instance, *patri badu* becomes *patri batu* and so on. In Sanskrit, an adolescent male came to be known as *vatu* at a later period and thus the word drifted a little away from the etymological meaning. The young *brahamachari*, however, is now also called *vatu* in Sanskrit. From the above analysis it is clear that *vatu*, which in Oriya is pronounced as *batu* and in colloquial Oriya as *badu*, primarily means 'bound to a particular kind of service', and in this sense *batu nritya* is a kind of ritual dance performed regularly in the Jagannatha temple at Puri. This surmise is corroborated by the inscription on the Jayavijaya *dvara* where the consecrated danseuses are designated as *bandha nachuni.*

Batu nritya which was being danced by the *bandha machunis* (i.e. the *maharis*) had in its repertoire both pure dance (*nritta*) and expressional dance (*nritya*) items. Since it was ritual dancing, it differed, more in content and spirit than in style for the performance at the royal court by dancers of professional calibre, and had a repertoire of both pure dance and expressional numbers.

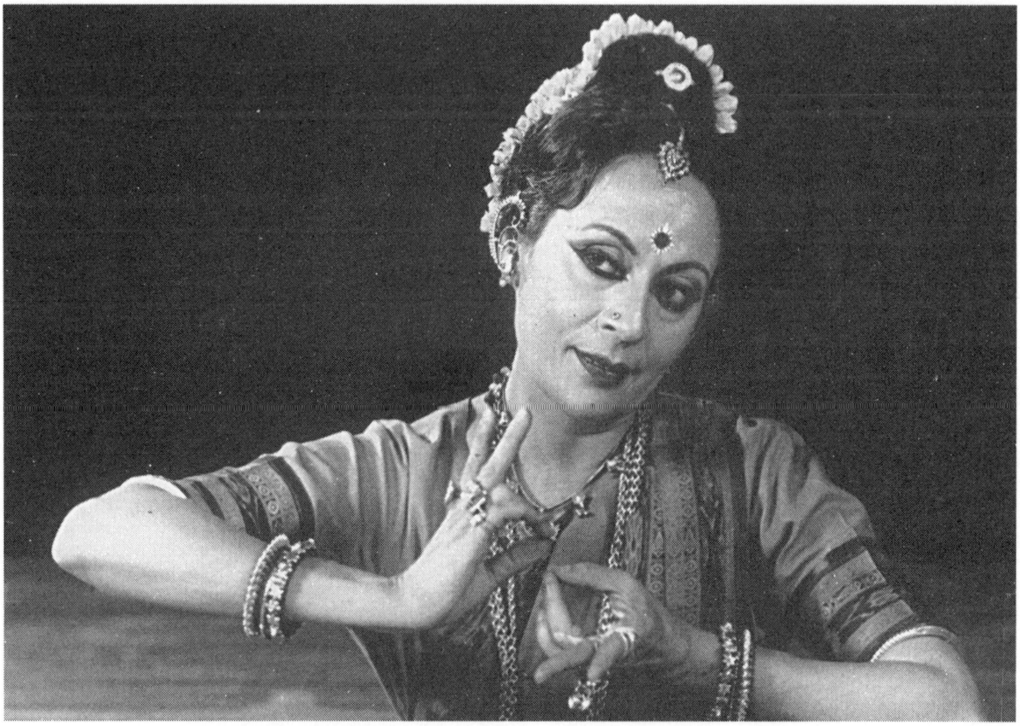

16. Sonal Mansingh, famous Odissi dancer presenting the *Shringara Bhava* through her dances. Photo: SNA, New Delhi.

Now the Odissi dancers present *batu* just after the invocatory *mangalacharana.* What they dance now used to be called *thayinata* (the local version of *sthayi nritya*), till the later part of the 1950s. Even today in some parts of rural Orissa, it is called *thayinaata*. One of the eminent living Odissi *gurus*, Debaprasad Das, does not call this number *batu*, but prefers to call it *sthayi nritya*.

Ballad Singing Traditions of Orissa

THE 'BALLAD' AS a song form is prevalent almost all over India. Some of the well-known forms are: *Pamdvani* of Madhya Pradesh, *Powada* of Maharashtra, *Alha* of Uttar Pradesh, *Heer-Ranjha* of Punjab, *Charan-geet* of Rajasthan, and so on. Orissa has several styles of ballad singing, of which two are more fascinating: *Pala* and *Daskathia* of which the former is more sophisticated.

Pala

This is a unique form of ballad singing that aesthetically blends elements of theatre, classical Odissi music, highly sophisticated Oriya and Sanskrit poetry with wit and humour. Usually, there are six to seven performers in a group of *pala* singers. It cannot be traditionally presented with less than four performers. The lead singer is called *gana* (also *gayaka*), the percussionist is called *bana* who plays a two-faced drum called *mrudanga*, and two to five associate singers called *palias* of which the leading one is called *shreepalia*. The ordinary *palas* play large cymbals called *kartal*.

Pala is presented in three ways: in the *baithaki pala* all the performers sit on the ground throughout; in the *thia pala*, which is more popular and aesthetically more satisfying, the performers stand while performing. The *badi pala* is a kind of *thia pala* in which there are two groups which vie with each other for excellence in performance. This last kind is the most entertaining, as there is an element of competition.

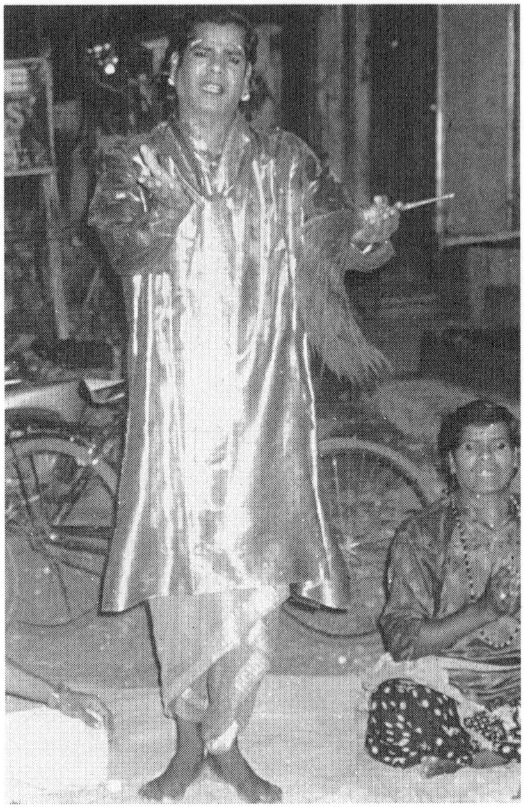

17. A *pala-gayak* presenting the performance with a *chaamar.* Photo: Dillip Tripathy.

A loud percussion ensemble, comprising the drum and large cymbals, precedes the singing. In this *gana*, the lead singer does not participate. The purpose of the percussion ensemble is twofold: to let the prospective audience know that the *pala* is going to be presented soon and the other is to serve as an aesthetic prelude (*poorva-ranga*). In the rural areas, the audience comes to the performance after dinner. Therefore, it usually begins around 8.30 or 9 p.m.

At the end of the musical prelude, the *gana* enters into the arena. Usually, it is on the level ground over which a large cotton made carpet is spread. The leading singer holds a flywhisk, called *chaamar*, in his hands, which he uses in different ways at different times. He begins with an invocation eulogizing the presiding deity. Traditionally, the *pala* is associated with the worship of Satyapeer, the deity that is accepted by both the Hindus and the Muslims. This trend can be traced back to the Mughal period when there was conscious efforts to bring about amity between the two religious faiths. After the invocation the *pala* proper begins. As in *daskathia* so also in *pala* the ballad is structured by the *gana* himself, but the style of structuring differs. The major portions of the *pala* ballad are stanzas of highly ornate Oriya poems written by eminent poets between seventeenth and fourth decade of twentieth century. The poems and *kavyas* (long narrative poems) written during this period were meant not only to be read but also to be sung in the *chhanda* styles of various kinds. The *gana* while structuring a particular *pala* ballad follows the same pattern as that of the classical Oriya *kavyas*. A *kavya* in its initial phase poetically narrates the birth of the hero and the heroine. Different cantos describe their growing up through the phases of infancy, adolescence, and youth. They meet and fall in love. Finally they marry. One or more cantos describe the beauty of the hero and especially, the heroine in each phase of their growing up. The description of the beauty of the heroine from head to toes at her youthful phase is given in great detail with wonderful similes. The *pala* ballad has the same structure. The description of the various aspects of her/his beauty are not written by the *gana* but is taken directly from the *kavyas* of different poets. For instance, the *pala* writer wants to describe the beauty of the eyes of a youthful heroine. He can take different relevant stanzas from various *kavyas* written either in Oriya or Sanskrit and attribute them all to the heroine of the *pala*. Thus borrowing from various poets the description of the beauty of the heroine's eye may go on for hours. The *gana* not only sings their stanzas in appropriate *chhanda* style, but also explains the meaning of the highly ornate lines in simple language. Thus through the *pala* sophisticated poetry was being popularized among common people. If the *gana* is not talented enough to structure a *pala* ballad, he may requisition the services of a suitable literary person to structure it for him. But he has to have an extraordinary memory to remember all the countless stanzas and a high degree of literary sensibility so that he can properly explain the meaning as well as the poetic merit to the common people. The singer who accepts to participate in a *badi pala* has indeed a phenomenal memory and ready wit, because the other singer may challenge him on any aspect of the *pala*.

The *gana* is also an excellent actor. While singing or explaining he brings in dramatic acting to heighten the appeal. He then uses his flywhisk as different properties. At one time it is used as the thunderbolt of god Indra, another time it may delineate the lyrical movement of waves and yet at another time the contour of a graceful creeper. He usually wears a costume similar to the formal dress of the erstwhile royal mobility. The others in the group wear also a kind of costume, which is not so splendid.

The role of the *palias* is, more or less, like the chorus boys. They sing the refrain of the song together with the *gana* and echo the last few words of the other sung lines. The role of *shreepalia* is of great importance in the performance as it is he who frequently interacts with the *gana* and punctuates the performance with wit and humour.

It is unfortunate that this unique, fascinating, and dignified tradition of performing art is gradually disappearing, because the people are so addicted to the popular mass media that the number of persons, who would prefer a *pala* performance to a film or a television serial, are very few. To be a good *gana*, besides multifaceted talent, one has to devote years of study and practice. It has to be a full time job. If one is not assured that the earning from this profession can make a decent living why one will be tempted to master this difficult art? The last great *ganas* were Harinath and Niranjan. They were in great demand till the early 1950s. The demand grew less and less, but there were sporadic *pala* performances till mid 1960s. Both are no longer there. None has come up who has even a fraction of their talent and excellence. Those groups who perform *pala* now are not even a shadow of the real art. They are at best amateurs, far from the excellence of a professional *pala* singer.

Daskathia

This is a fascinating form of ballad singing that admirably blends elements of theatre, music, wit and humour. It is, however, not as sophisticated as *pala*. *Daskathia* requires only two singer actors for the performance, the duration of which may be from around two hours to eight hours, that is, the whole night, depending upon the audience and the theme of the ballad. The main singer is called *gayaka*. He is assisted by the *palia*. Both of them play a kind of castanets called *daskathi* from which the form has derived its name. The *gayaka* plays a bigger and different kind of castanets and it has also another name: *ramtali*. The *gayaka* plays it sparingly. It is the *palia* who is an expert in playing the smaller pair of castanets called *daskathi*. He punctuates the performance with percussion music of highly complex and fascinating rhythmic passages. He also punctuates with passages of wit and humor that enhances the appeal of the performance.

Thus, the importance of the *palia* is no less than the main singer. The *gayaka* must have very good voice, because it is he who sings the entire ballad and the *palia* echoes only the last one or two words of the sung line.

The singing style is, more or less, in accordance with the *chhanda* form of Odissi classical music. The themes of the ballads are usually drawn from the vast body of Indian mythological literature, especially those, which have Oriya versions. Invariably the *gayaka* himself composes the ballad in verse form taking interesting episodes from the mythology. The *gayaka* not only sings but also explains and elaborates in imromptu prose. He wears a costume that is similar to what the erstwhile rulers were wearing on formal occasions.

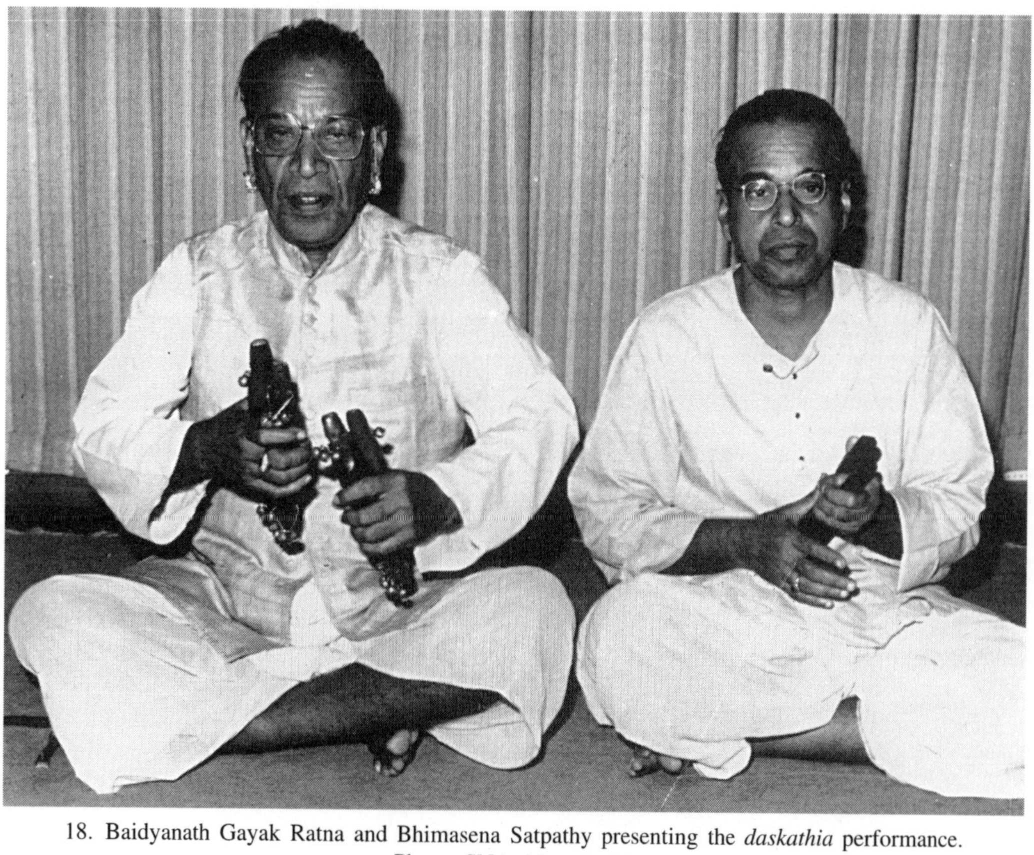

18. Baidyanath Gayak Ratna and Bhimasena Satpathy presenting the *daskathia* performance. Photo: SNA, New Delhi.

In *daskathia* the vocal music of the *gayaka* is accompanied with the percusion music of the castanets. No other musical instrument is used in this form of ballad singing.

Although, *daskathia* originated in the southern part of Orissa, especially in the district of Ganjam, it has now spread to the other parts. More *daskathia* singers are still in the Ganjam district.

Tradition and Innovation in Odissi

As in Sanskrit so also in Oriya and a few other Indian languages, tradition is called *parampara* that literally means 'after and after'. It unmistakably suggests continuous change. *Parampara* therefore is a flow like a river that takes not only several turns, but also several tributary inflows. Conservatives, however, think that *parampara* is an accumulation like a lake and individual talents are like showers that raise its level. In fact, individual talents and influences are like tributaries that increase the quality and quantity of the *parampara* flow. The concept of innovation is inherent in *parampara*. The inflows, that is, the influences and innovations should enrich the flow, not pollute it or change its basic character. Only then does *parampara* grow and maintain its aesthetic qualities. In this perspective, let us examine the contemporary innovations and the quality of *parampara* flow during the last five decades.

Several treatises on Odissi dance written between sixteenth and nineteenth centuries and countless other references point to the fact that three classes of dancers were performing this style of dance. The dance of the *maharis* in the temple was basically ritualistic. The *nartakis* danced in the royal courts and for the general public in traditional festivals like Vasantotsava (Spring festival). Their dance primarily aimed at imparting aesthetic relish (*rasanubhuti*) to the audience. From around the sixteenth century, another class of dancers called *gotipua* began to perform the dance for the masses. Their dance was aesthetically satisfying, but with a touch of popular appeal. Owing to extreme change in social values and gradual withdrawal of royal patronage, the *nartakis* were the first to disappear from the scene by around latter half of nineteenth century. The *maharis* continued to dance in the temple of Lord Jagannatha at Puri till the fourth decade of the twentieth century, but their dance had decayed so much that it was more ritual than dance. The last recognized *mahari* was known as Kunda Mahari. Those who are now being paraded as *maharis* were not recognized dancing *maharis* and their names are not found in the temple register. It is the *gotipua* class of dancers who continued the tradition, but their dance had become so full of popular appeal that the classicism of the dance was diluted. In the year 1959, some scholars and a few *gurus* came together and cleansed the dance of its decadent trends with the help of dance treatises and temple sculptures. The present repertoire of Odissi is, more or less, what this group of scholars and *gurus* formed.

Odissi for centuries had been a Solo dance. Now under the name of innovation, group performances of Odissi are being presented. The word choreography is now so much used that one gets bewildered by it. Choreography is basically a Western concept. I am not against the inroad of the concept into the field of Indian classical dance. But the concept behind the word must be first understood and then brought in, in such a way that it does not distort the classicism or character of the dance style. Most of the group Odissi dances can be easily termed as Solo multiples. Now even the intra-form called *mangalacharan* (often the invocatory number) is presented as a group performance. The so-called choreographer perhaps does not understand the difference between *mangalacharan* and an *abhinaya* number based on a devotional song. While the former is iconogrpahic in character, performed as *poorva-ranga*, the latter is expressional, that aims at giving an aestheic experience to the audience. Most of the Odissi *gurus* do not have any theoretical knowledge and therefore have little idea of dance aesthetics. The dance lovers are also equally ignorant. Therefore, they gladly gulp whatever is glamorous and offbeat. A group presentation of *mangalacharan* is neither innovation nor Odissi.

In defence of the so-called choreographers, I would like to point out that this trend of presenting Solo multiples, not only in Odissi but also in other classical dance styles, is so rampant because in India we do not have a single theatre hall which is suitable for Solo dancing. The proscenium stage may be all right for presenting a play, but most unsuitable for Solo classical dances in which expressional numbers are very important because only these give the audience a taste of the *rasa*. In a hall with a proscenium stage, the spectators sitting beyond the first few rows can hardly see the subtle facial expressions. Again, the stage is so big that the Solo dancer appears almost as a miniature dynamic figurine. In order to cover the large dancing area she moves much more than she should. These two (of the many) disadvantages of the proscenium stage have prompted the dance *gurus* to compose group numbers and pass them off as innovations.

In the obscure past some individual talent must have innovated the intraform called *pallavi*. The innovation not only fitted beautifully in the grammar and style of the dance but also enhanced its aesthetic quality. Therefore, the connoiseurs of that time accepted it as Odissi and other dancers started composing *pallavis* in different *ragas*. It was then accepted as an intraform in the traditional repertoire of Odissi dance. Such innovations are most welcome, but not the hybridized ones, which may be modern dance but certainly not Odissi.

From this perspective all the multiplied Solo compositions and innovative choreographic presentations can be classed under one category: the modern dance. To innovate within the framework of a particular classical dance *paramparas* requires genius of highest degree. The *parampara* is a flow, but not just any flow. For instance flood is also a flow. It may have a tremendous personality, but no *character*. Whereas the flow of a river has both personality as well as character. The two banks of a river give it its character. In a classical dance *parampara*, its grammar, aesthetic consideration, and mode of presentation, form the banks. The innovation should be a tributary to the *parampara* so that it can merge itself in the flow. The innovation in a particular style of dance that cannot flow with the *parampara* is like a sandy shore on beside of the flow. The shore may be very beautiful and sparkling with golden grains, but it cannot merge itself into the flow. Thus during the last fifty years there have been many innovations some of which may be very impressive, but most of them are not *paramparik* innovations. The few dancers who have done Solo innovations without being influenced by the Western trends have not received media attention to the desired extent. As a result, choreographers are increasingly copying the West and gradually drifting away from *parampara*.

How many Indians know the deep and poetic symbolism behind our rituals and mythology? Have we not transformed our *dharma* into a religion and politicians take advantage of this? Is it not time after, more than fifty years of our independence that we should regain our distinctive 'Indianness'?

Krishna in Indian Dance

KRISHNA IS MORE A concept than a character. He is not merely a male but the male principle. Again, even if Krishna was a historical person, as a mythological figure or a mystical symbol he transcended the temporal plane. The basic difference between history and mythology is that while the former tells of things part, the latter tells simultaneoulsy of past, present and future.

Deep in the mists of time, the myth of Krishna and Radha began 'thinking' in the minds of the Ahirs, a highly cultured non-Aryan tribe. In fact, 'Aryan' is a synthesized culture that integrated many diverse ones to form a unified whole. When a culture lent itself to integration, it did so perhaps with the understanding that its myths and its gods were also appropriately assimilated. Of the several 'non-Aryan' cultures which willingly merged with the broadbased Aryan culture, those of the Ahirs and the Shavaras were among the most developed. While the Ahir culture gave Krishna and Radha to the Aryan pantheon, the Shavara culture gave Jagannatha. Although Krishna got ready acceptance as a God and by the fourth century BC he was regarded as Vasudeva (son of Vasudeva) Radha had to wait till about the sixth century AD when the *Brahmavaivarta Purana* is believed to have been written, for entering the Aryan mythology as an important deity. Since then Krishna and Radha have been 'thinking' in the minds of the Hindus. By the twelfth century, when the two were not only 'thinking' but were singing mellifluously in the mind of the poet Jayadeva, they had touched the deepest depth of the human mind as infinitely complex symbols. During the sixteenth century when Krishna and Radha were active in the minds of Chaitanya Deva and his friends and followers they were not only concepts and symbols but also mystic experiences. Throughout, the history of their 'thinking' in men, Radha and Krishna have remained basically the symbols of the totality of Love which is as vast as infinity.

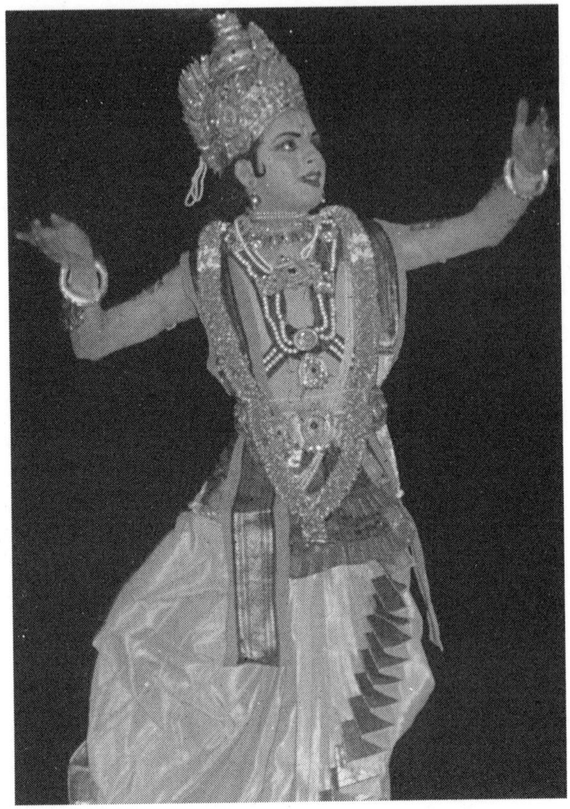

19. Venket Subramanyam Prasad in the role of Krishna, presenting the Kuchipudi dance. Photo: SNA, New Delhi.

Right from the beginning of creation, two forces are acting on us: Ego and Love. While Ego is the separative force, Love is the unifying one; and each has a perspective. From the perspective of the Ego, the created universe is an endless diversity, but from that of the Love, it is one. Krishna is the symbol of Love, the unifying force, which has again two aspects, one that is sweet (*madhurya*) and the other that is majestic (*aishvarya*). Radha is the symbol of the sweet aspect of Love, while Rukmini and Satyabhama, are symbols of the glamorous aspect. Both aspects have been admirably developed in Indian mythology. Owing to its inherent impressive character, the majestic aspect is dramatic whereas the sweet aspect is lyrical and poetic.

The relationship of Krishna with Rukmini or Satyabhama is not as complex as with Radha. In the former case, if both are reduced from concepts to characters (i.e. from mythological perspective to that of historical) nothing is lost, but if Krishna and Radha are reduced to mere 'characters', the whole issue gets highly distorted. The Vaishnavas have given several analogies to explain the highly complex and infinitely subtle relationship between Radha and Krishna, of which the oft-cited one is the relationship between *madhu* (sugar, literally honey) and *madhurata* (sweetness). Sugar without sweetness is meaningless. Sweetness is contained in sugar while sugar is expressed through sweetness; they are inseparable. Conceptionally, one is separated from the other only to comprehend the function of each. This has been very subtly indicated by Jayadeva in the seventh *ashtapadi* of the *Geetagovinda* beginning with the words: *maamiyam chalita vilokya*. In the sixth couplet of the *ashtapadi* Krishna says, 'If I am ever united with Radha, why am I searching for her in this forest?' Yet he goes on looking for her. The answer to Krishna's question is the reason behind his *leela* which is spread from the temporal plane to the mystic. If these two planes are conceived as two poles of eternity then Radha and Krishna have two separate forms (*rupas*). At the mystic plane, the duo is inseparably united and that is the eternal form (*nityarupa*). At the plane bound by time and space, they appear as two separate entities aspiring for union and that is the temporal form (*leelarupa*). They perform the *leela* only to enable the human mind to comprehend the ultimate reality of the *nityarupa*.

It is not difficult to identify Krishna with God and consider the mythological figure as only a symbol. It is not, however, at all easy to comprehend the complexity and subtlety of the Radha symbol. She represents the long but continuous stretch from matter to spirit. Except the mystics, no one until the early decades of the twentieth century could imagine that matter to energy is but a continuous stretch and each can be approached from the other's side. The nuclear scientists have proved beyond doubt that matter can be converted into energy and vice-versa. But even the scientists do not know what is spirit although they cannot deny its existence. Therefore, with the rational mind, it is impossible to comprehend the whole stretch from matter to spirit. One has to have a poet's awareness which, following the famous French poet Rimbud's prescription, has undergone a reasoned derangement of senses, to comprehend a little of Radha's entire stretch.

The concept is so complex that the symbol (that is, the mythological character) could not be simpler; Radha is a unique blending of (i) a woman deeply in love with the divine, (ii) a devotee, (iii) a housewife (that is, a social being), (iv) an unceasing aspiration for merging her identity with that of the divine, (v) the materialized form of primal energy that makes the divine dynamic and creative, and (vi) a total human being who at times is influenced by the Ego.

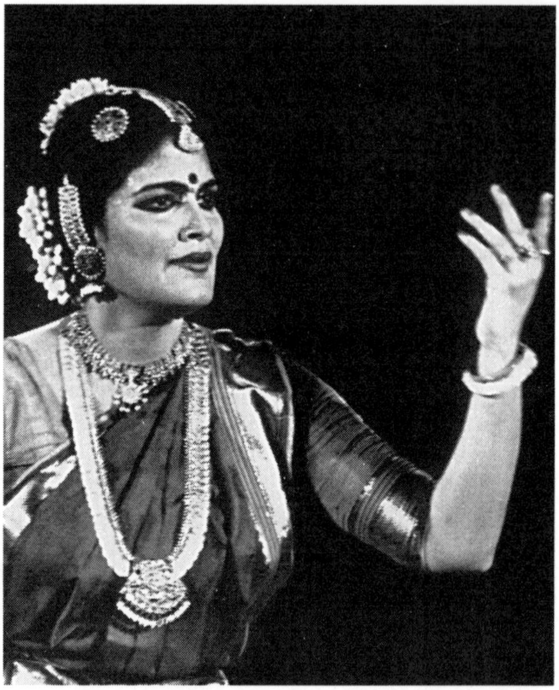

20. Gita Chandran performing the Bharatanatyam. Photo: SNA, New Delhi.

Since Ego is the separative force, when Radha is influenced by it she feels separated from Krishna and is in anguish. The introductory *shloka* to the third *ashtapadi* of *Geetagovinda* (*lalita lavangalata parisheelana*) poetically describes this anguished state of Radha. For understanding the relationship between Radha and Krishna in this state, let us take this line from Kabir's writing, *Jala me kumbha aur kumbha me jala hai bhitar bahar paani* (the pitcher is inside water and water is inside the pitcher and both outside and inside the pitcher is water). The meaning of this deeply poetic and metaphysical line can be comprehended if you imagine a pitcher, after being filled up with water, sunk to the bottom of the sea. The pitcher thinks that her heart is full of the sea. Similarly, the sea thinks that he is holding the pitcher in his heart. If the pitcher under the influence of Ego becomes too possessive, she will feel jealous and anguished when she sees that other pitchers filled with the same sea water are sinking down towards the bottom of the sea. This is the condition of Radha when she beholds Krishna dancing with other *gopis*. Jayadeva in his *Geetagovinda* describes in mellifluous poetry the successive stages of Radha's journey towards the divine, shedding at each stage some amount of the Ego's influence. When she is totally liberated from the Ego, both the devotee and the divine become one experience, in which identity of each merges with that of the other.

As characters, Radha and Krishna live in the mythical reality which is much larger than life and therefore appears non-real. For elucidation, let us take an example. A very thin chip of the stem of a plant may appear to the naked eye as a translucent greenish-white small disc. When it is seen through a powerful microscope it presents a totally different picture. Many hundred times magnified, it reveals the beautiful structure of its cells. Or, an artist may draw a picture of the chip. Here then, are three versions of a reality: the chip seen by the naked eye is true to life; what is observed through the microscope is larger than life; the painting is the artistic reality which appears non-realistic since it depicts the larger-than-life picture. When Radha and Krishna are appropriately portrayed on the stage the third kind of reality is usually presented to the audience. If the portrayal, however, becomes true to life, then the two are no longer Radha and Krishna, but a pair of human lovers not much different form the hero and heroine as they appear in any ordinary dramatic presentation.

The traditional Indian theatre and classical dance styles are deliberately highly stylized because they were appropriately shaped to handle mythical reality, so that the performance gave a much deeper aesthetic satisfaction, together with a better understanding of the infinite complexities of life.

It is significant to note that traditional Indian thinking could never conceive of a serious theatre without the predominance of dance elements. A line in *Harivamsa* says, *naatakam nartayitu* which means a play should be danced. Again, the Sanskrit word for theatre is *natya* which is derived from the root *nat*, meaning to dance. The elements of dance not only give the Indian art of acting, *abhinaya*, a choreographic character, but also impart to the performance a good deal of theatrical power to handle easily dramatic situations much larger than life. In fact, theatre traditions like Kutiyattam, Krishnattam and Kathakali of Kerala, have so much of the dance element that Westerners think Kathakali is a dance style rather than theatre. Like Krishnattam of Kerala, Rasaleela of the Braj region is exclusivley based on Krishna legend. While the former deals with the *aishvarya* aspect of Krishna, the latter with the *madhurya*. In Rasaleela, however music dominates the dance elements, but it is also highly stylized, to handle the *madhurya* aspect.

All Indian classical dances draw heavily upon the Krishna legend. Manipuri has been inspired exclusively by its *madhurya* aspect. Many expressional numbers in the traditional repertoire of Kathak, Odissi, Bharatanatyam and Kuchipudi are based on poems inspired by it. In fact, Kuchipudi was originally a theatre form dealing with the *aishvarya* aspect. The Solo dancing in the said styles present the legend in yet another aesthetic dimension. The dancer in the same costume portrays through highly stylized gestural *abhinaya*, Krishna, Radha a *gopi* or any other character in the legend and therefore it is called *ekaharya* type of *abhinaya*. This is a unique kind of performance in which the Solo dancer with his or her histrionic talent and gestural acting populates the danced dimension.

It is however, to be admitted that most of these rich and unparalleled traditions of theatre and dance under the strong influence of alien cultures started acquiring decadent tendencies, because dance, which was regarded in India as one of the most suitable expressions for delineation of the spiritual experience, gradually became a means for entertainment. In some feudal courts dance was pulled down to the level where it functioned only as a stimulant for passion. In a feudalistic society invariably the subjects adopt the value pattern of the ruler. Therefore, what the general audience wanted from a dancer was not much different from the feudal lords. The situation, of course, changed with the political independence of this country. But have we attained mental and intellectual independence, or are we still suffering from a strong colonial hangover? If we are changing, are we becoming more Indian or poor imitators of Western culture? It is high time that we answer the question truthfully and decide upon our future course of action.

Under the prevailing circumstances very few dancers perhaps know the difference between the Radha-Krishna duo and the hero-heroine duo of the Indian film industry! Therefore, the desire to see the duo delineated as one, while maintaining the symbolic depth, may not be easily satisfied now.

From the seventeenth century onwards, social esteem for dance became so low that even during the early decades of the present century it was the preserve of a special kind of entertainer. A saying aptly sums up the social attitude of a certain section of people towards dance, 'One who has some elements of shame plays only a musical instrument, one with none, sings, but one who is extremely shameless, dances.'

The climate changed to some extent from the 1950s and soon dancing became a fashion. Many of the classical dancers now behave more like film stars than genuine artistes. Exceptions only prove my point of view. And what about the *gurus*? Because of the adverse social attitude towards dancing, those who were taking to it as profession were not provided with opportunities conducive to their vocation, nor were they adequately educated to understand the complexity and subtlety of our dance traditions. The dance *gurus*, again barring very few exceptions, may be well versed in the techniques of dance, but they did not have any idea of the aesthetics, nor did they have the intellectual equipment to comprehend the difference between the physical reality and mythical reality. Therefore, they taught their disciples how to dance with the body alone, leaving the mind pedestrian. As a result, Radha and Krishna are often portrayed in our classical dances as earthy creatures with a strong passion, or as a frail bundle of sentiments. And what about the general audience? For most of them, the ideal entertainment is a commercial movie.

In such a climate which is so heavily dominated by film culture, Radha and Krishna would surely feel suffocated. That is why they are still hiding inside our glorious mythology, waiting for the day when India will achieve freedom from the clutch of the merchants of entertainment.

Krishna in Kathak

Kathak, right from its initial phase of development, has been deeply associated with Krishna legend. The earliest mention of Kathak as an art is found in the *Arjuna-vanavasa* chapter of the *adi-parva* of the *Mahabharata.* From this reference it is evident that Kathak was in its initial phase a kind of mimetic recitation of Puranic literature, most probably embellished with dance passages. Kaiyata of tenth century AD, while writing a commentary on the *Mahabhashya* of Patanjali, says that the Kathakas are but Granthikas who were known for reciting stories related to Vishnu. Naturally, when Krishna was identified with Vishnu, the Granthika, i.e. the Kathak, a must have begun telling the stories of Krishna. Scholars believe that in the Mathura region, a rich tradition of performing arts, especially *natya*, developed during the early centuries. It may be mentioned here that the belt where the Ahirs used to live comprise the areas now known as Uttar Pradesh, Rajasthan, Gujarat and Maharashtra.

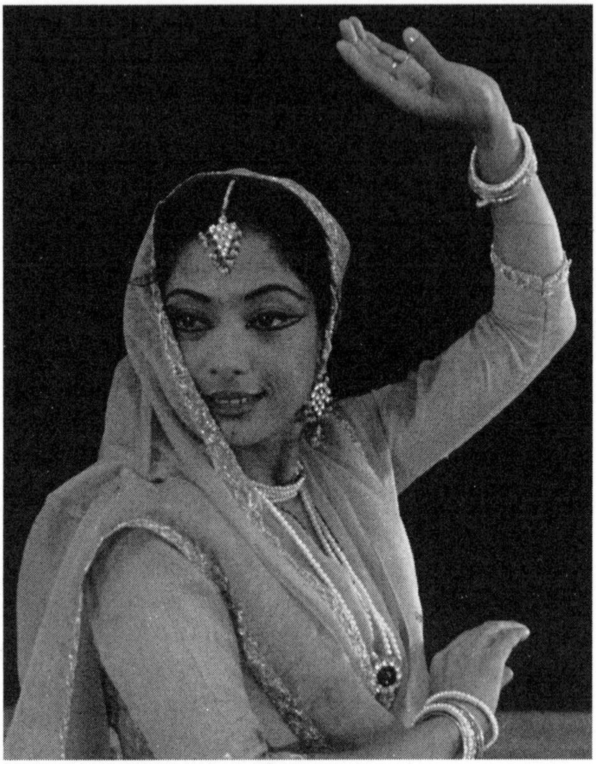

21. Saswati Sen in Kathak postures.
Photo: SNA, New Delhi.

Scholars also believe that the Kathak dance has an unmistakable relation with Rasaleela, which is a musical theatre form evidently grown out of the rich Krishnaite theatre tradition of the Mathura region. It may, therefore, be surmised that up to the fifteenth century the art of *katha vaachan*, which is the earliest form of Kathak, was exclusively based on Krishna legend. The *katha vaachan* that now survives, though much emaciated, in a few places near Mathura and Vrindavan, deals exclusively with the Krishna stories. During the sixteenth century the art of Kathak started coming to royal courts from the temple precincts and the seventeenth century it received strong patronage from both Hindu and Mughal feudals.

At the royal courts, the art of Kathak acquired a good deal of secular element and sophistication, especially in the pure dance passages. At this phase of its development Kathak drew inspiration increasingly from percussion music. The anklebells tied to a dancer's feet became more and more articulate and the pure dance items began to be so structured as to recreate the percussion music both aurally and visually. This development imparted to the dance style a sparkling character and required the dancer to be a virtuoso through long and arduous practice. The initial element of story telling gave way to expressional dancing, more often steeped in romantic fervour.

At this period of time under the influence of alien cultures, dancing, which in India was mostly regarded as a form of worship or artistic activity of a very high order, started being considered more as entertainment aimed at appealing to the sensual appeal of their singing. A large number of songs, especially *Thumris* written on the love theme of Krishna and Radha, were interpreted by the courtesans. This trend continued till the early decades of twentieth century. Although a large number of Kathak performers were courtesans, their teachers were invariably male dancers who used to present the expressional passages based on the Krishna-Radha love theme with great subtlety and delicacy. A few of these male dancers, like Maharaj Bindadin, used to get generous patronage from the feudals.

In Indian mythology, two divinities are regarded as great dancers, Lord Shiva, the Nataraj; and Lord Krishna, the Natavara. Dancing, the Nataraj is predominantly of *tandava* type, that of the Natavara is of *lasya* type. Many eminent Kathak dancers of recent past were of the firm opinion that the Kathak dance evolving from the dancing of Lord Krishna should be named Natavari. Even now a few prefer to call the dance style Natavari Kathak rather than simply Kathak. In their opinion the art of *katha vaachan* should appropriately be called Kathak, but the classical dance style that grew out of it should be Natavari. Whether the dance style is called Kathak or Natavari, there is no doubt that it has a deep association with the Krishna legend down the centuries and for enhancing its aesthetic appeal the association with the Krishna legend should be made more deep, not from the perspective of religion but from that of poetic sensibilities, by emphasizing the mystical and metaphysical symbolism it acquired through the concept of *madhura-bhakti.*

Kavitt—The Poetry of Dance

IN ITS INITIAL PHASE of development, Kathak was a mimetic art (*abhinaya-pradhan*). From the seventeenth century, it became *tala pradhan*. This major deviation resulted in the inclusion of many new intraforms in the Kathak repertoire. One can confidently surmise that intraforms such as *tukda salami*, *aamad*, *gatnikaas* and so on came in after the turn. But such intraforms as *kavitt, paran* and *tatkaar* are perhaps not so new, although they might have undergone considerable modifications after the turn.

Kavitt, like *kavita*, literally means poetry. The former is in masculine form whereas the latter feminine. But in Kathak *kavitt* denotes a certain kind of brief dance number structured on a particular kind of verbal composition. The composition has two components (*anga*), meaningful words and (*sahitya*) mixed with meaningless words which are but mnemonic syllables (*pata*) pertaining mainly to *tabla* and *pakhawaj*.

The tradition of singing mnemonic syllables for various musical instruments is very old in India. It was prevalent even in the days of the *Natya Shastra*. Such renderings were then known as *bahirgeet* or *nirgeet*. In the *Prabandha* singing, which is the precursor of *Dhruvapada* (Dhrupad), musical rendering of the mnemonic syllables (*paata-gayan*) was one of the six *angas* (components). The six *angas* are *pada*, verse or poem with meaningful words; *virulla*, eulogy of the presiding being of the *Prabandhas*; *tala*, the time measure; *svara*, solfa passages; *patta*, the mnemonic syllables; and *tenaka* auspicious words like *tena*, *nana* and so on. *Prabandhas* using two, three, four, five and all the six *angas* were categorized respectively under *taravali*, *bhavani*, *deepani*, *anandini* and *medini*.

When *Prabandha* singing went out of vogue, giving way first to *Dhruvapada* and then to *Khayal*, most probably the *deepani* category of *Prabandha* inspired the singing of *chaturanga*, literally means 'having four components'. These *angas* are: *pada*, also called *sahitya*; *svara*, solfa passages; *tarana*, singing of meaningless syllables; and *trivat*, singing of mnemonic syllables pertaining to *pakhawaj*.

The *Bhavani* category of *Prabandha* with three *angas* was rendered with *pada*, *tala*, and either *svara* or *pata*. *Kavitt* too has three *angas*: *pada*, *tala* and *pata*. It is therefore worth-while to compare the two so that the aesthetic objective of *kavitt* becomes clear.

In *Bhavani*, the *pada* part was surely sung as in *chaturanga*, which means that greater importance was laid on the rendering of the *raga* in which the *sahitya* was couched. However, in *kavitt* the *sahitya* is not sung but rendered in a recitative style. When the meaningful word does not soar on the wings of a *raga* but swings on the waves of a *tala*, it has to carry more poetic charge so that the aesthetic appeal does not flag. The poetic quality of a lyric written to be sung essentially differs from that of a poem meant to be recited. The mnemonic syllables used in a *Bhavani Prabandha* were either sung or rhythmically recited as is now done in a *pallavi* composition in Odissi dance (*pallavis* also have three *angas* namely *pata*, *svara*, and *tala* with no *pada*). In the *kavitt*, however, the *pada* and *pata* are interwoven to form a united whole. Therefore, the *pata* phrases should aim at appropriately ornamenting the *pada* phrases so that the mimetic movements come out in high relief.

Evidently, *kavitt* comes under the expressional (*nritya*) category. According to traditional Indian thinking, expres-sional dance is visual poetry. Compared to a *padam* in Bharatanatyam or an *abhinaya* number in Odissi, *kavitt* is a very brief number. Although there are lengthy *kavitts*, their real character comes out when they are brief. A really well-done *kavitt* could therefore be described as visual haiku.

There are, of course, bad haiku; just as there are bad *kavitts*. Generally, dancers belonging to the Jaipur *gharana* now present *kavitts*. Dancers of the Lucknow *gharana* seldom include a *kavitt* in their recitals now, though there are quite a few in their *gharana's* repertoire. Unfortunately, most of the *kavitts* presented nowadays are weak in their aesthetic appeal, mainly because they are performed in a tempo faster than *madhya laya* (medium pace). As a result, the mimetic aspect gets totally blurred and it appears more like a *nritta* than a *nritya* item. Watching these *kavitts* performed in the *barabar laya* is somewhat like watching a film running in the projector at double the normal speed. Once I persuaded Nandini Singh to perform the *kavitts* at a much slower tempo and the result was satisfying as it was bound to be. Guru Munnalal Shukla gives me to understand that Lachhu Maharaj, who composed a number of beautiful *kavitts*, always insisted that they be performed in a much slower tempo.

It is not easy to compose the verbal layout of a *kavitt*. For, in effect, it requires the talent of a good haiku writer combined with the sensitivity and creativity of a musician who has a complete command over *layakari*. It does not end there. When the verbal material is ready, it requires a highly economic choreographer to give the composition an artistic visual form. In lesser hands *kavitts* may sound ridiculous even if they are executed skilfully. The dancers who perform such funny-sounding *kavitts* should understand that dance is as much for the eyes as for the ears.

It is also worthwhile to compare the *kavitt* with the few *parans* named after some of the deities, such as, Ganeshaparan, Lakshmiparan and so on. The verbal composition of these *parans* bears much similarity to the *kavitts*, but if their execution is carefully watched, it will be evident that they figure more under *nritta* than under *nritya*. There is a distinct difference between mimetic and iconographic dance movements and gestures.

If a well-composed and tastefully executed *kavitt* is carefully watched, one will be convinced that this intraform existed in the storytelling phase of Kathak, perhaps in a different form. In all likelihood these short and intensely poetic *kavitts* punctuated the long narrative mime passages. Now, when Kathak is a classical dance form and no longer limited to 'storytelling', the *kavitts* have the potential to be much more interesting than the *tukdas* and *parans*—provided they are well composed both verbally and in terms of dance movements. Here in fact, is an area where the creative and innovative minds in the field of Kathak can contribute much to enrich and expand the repertoire, while well within the established parameters.

Bhav-batana is the most poetic and intensely dramatic of all the expressional passages in the tradition of Kathak. Unlike *gat-bhav* and *gat-nikas*, the *bhav-batana* passages are magnificently based on verbal material which may not be poetic at all. As the name suggests, the dancer indicates the *bhav* which is not there in the verbal words. *Bhav-batana* passages demand fabulous imagination from the dancer and a great command of gestural acting (*angikabhinaya*) so that intensely poetic suggestions are visually presented with highly economized and subtle movements of the limbs. The Kathak dancer who has reached the pinnacle of maturity is incapable of presenting *bhav-batana* in an inappropriate way! No wonder Ananda Coomaraswamy in the preface of the *Mirror of Gesture* (*Abhinaya Darpana*) says that the *bhav-batana* of Kathak is the *quintessence* of Indian *natya* tradition. It is indeed a pity that *bhav-batana* is now on the verge of extinction.

Indian Folk Theatre

INDIA HAS AN EXTREMELY rich and varied theatre tradition. The vast body of traditional theatre is basically classified into *Folk* and *Classical*. This dichotomy is not relevant to Indian theatre and dance. There are quite a few theatre styles, which have almost all the qualities of a so-called classical theatre. For instance, Krishnattam of Kerala and Rasaleela of Uttar Pradesh are highly developed forms of theatre. The singing of the *padas* of Rasaleela is like that of the Dhrupad. Krishnattam is the precursor of Kathakali. Although Kathakali is actually a form of theatre, it is now regarded as a form of classical dance. Each Kathakali play has a definite plot and development of characters. It may be a form of dance from the Western perspective. Dancing in Kathakali is one of the kinds of dramatic expression what Brecht calls 'choreographic acting'. In India, theatre could never be conceived without elements of music and dance. We call theatre *natya* that is derived from the verbal root of *nat*, which means 'to dance'. The only surviving classical Sanskrit theatre is Kutiyattam, which has almost all the aspects of Kathakali. Most of the theatre styles, which are being classified under the folk category, have elements of dance and music and have been inspired by the concept of *natya*, the Sanskrit theatre.

Nowadays all the serious theatre thinkers of the West seem to prefer total theatre to dialogue-centered realistic theatre. The total theatre has elements of poetry, music, dance, etc., and most of our theatre styles are, in a sense, total theatre. Therefore, it would be more appropriate to classify them as traditional language theatre rather than folk theatre.

In ancient India, Sanskrit was the *rashtrabhasha*, that is, the lingua franca of this country. All our great plays written even until the sixteenth century are in Sanskrit. When regional languages were fully developed, Sanskrit started receding from the common man. Therefore, theatre forms of various styles began evolving, using different regional languages, but their model was Sanskrit theatre. That is why the language theatre forms have elements of dance and music and they are, more or less stylized theatre forms.

Another interesting aspect of our language theatre forms is the highly stylized make-up and costumes, especially in south India. The Yakshgana of Karnataka, Therukoothu of Tamil Nadu, Mudiettu, Teyyam, and Padayani of Kerala, and Prahlada Nataka of Orissa use highly stylized make-up and costumes. In the Teyyam theatre of Kerala the actor's face

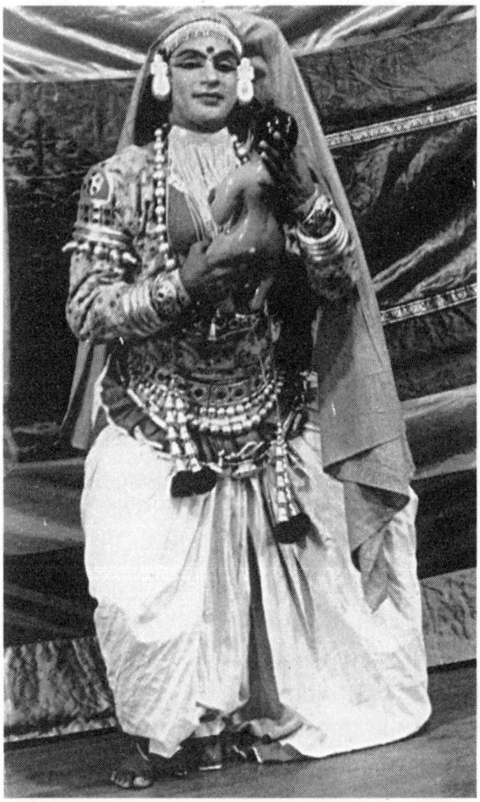

22. Putana Mokshyam performing by a Krishnattam dancer. Photo: SNA, New Delhi.

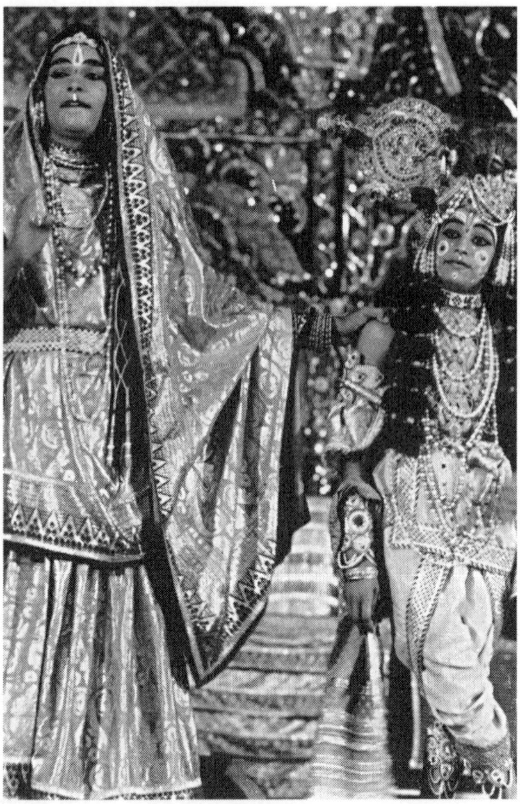

23. A scene from Rasaleela, Uttar Pradesh. Photo: SNA, New Delhi.

is treated with bright colours to give it a mask-like appearance and some of the actors wear such huge headgear that it may go up to 30 feet. To keep the headgear upright, a stagehand props it up with a bamboo pole. In Krishnattam many characters wear highly stylized make up and about eight of the characters wear wooden masks.

There is an aesthetic reason for such stylized make-up and costumes. It is to prevent the audience from identifying with the portrayed characters. Brecht, the great German playwright and theatre thinker, who has profoundly influenced the theatre persons all over the world suggests emphatically that the audience must be *alienated* from the portrayed characters on the stage so that he or she is dissuaded from any kind of identification, with dramatis personae. If any of the audience identifies himself or herself with any of the portrayed characters of the stage then he or she will have almost the same kind of mental state of the character, which will cloud the faculty of judgement. As a result, the onlooker will not clearly comprehend the moral of the theatrical presentation. The highly stylized make-up and costumes used in many of our language theatre forms are precisely devices for Brechtian 'alienation'.

Music is the life breath of many of our language theatre forms. The theatre music admirably blends folk with classical. Some of the highly musical language theatres are Kuchipudi theatre of Andhra Pradesh, Rasaleelas and Nautanki of Uttar Pradesh, Tamasha of Maharashtra, Jatra theatre of Orissa and Bengal, Ankianat of Assam, Bhavai of Gujarat, Khyal of Rajasthan and Mach of Madhya Pradesh.

In some of our language theatre forms, percussion is as powerful as it is dramatic. In Kathakali, the drum called *chende* wonderfully enhances the dramatic as well as the aesthetic quality. When a character is dreaming, the *chende* will be playing so softly and lyrically that its sound suggests dreaming. If however, there is a fight between two characters, the *chende* will be played with such fury that the intensity of the scene will be enhanced many times. The drum called *nakkara* is equally eloquent in Nautanki of Uttar Pradesh, *Swang* of Haryana, and Khyal of Rajasthan. These three theatre forms have similarities for which some scholars are of opinion that once upon a time they belonged to a theatre style called Sang which might have been inspired by the *sangeetaka uparoopaka* (musical sub-form) of Sanskrit theatre.

Almost all the language theatre forms are not realistic and dialogue-centred. They are deliberately theatrical and the dramatic situations are much larger than life. In quite a few language theatre forms, at times, dialogues are delivered in the form of songs. There is also very often exaggeration in expressing emotions, which may appear melodramatic, but that is the vitality of the theatre forms. The exaggeration is deliberateric aimed at heightening the theatricality. Those who are for realistic theatre they may dislike the theatricality,

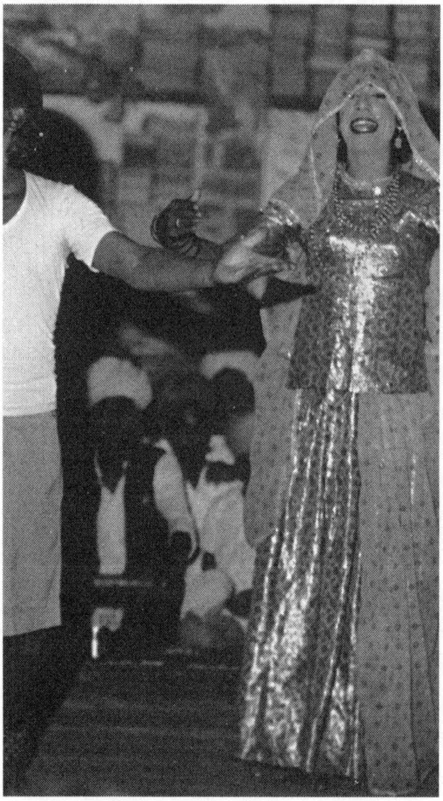

24. Khyal, Rajasthan. Photo: SNA, New Delhi.

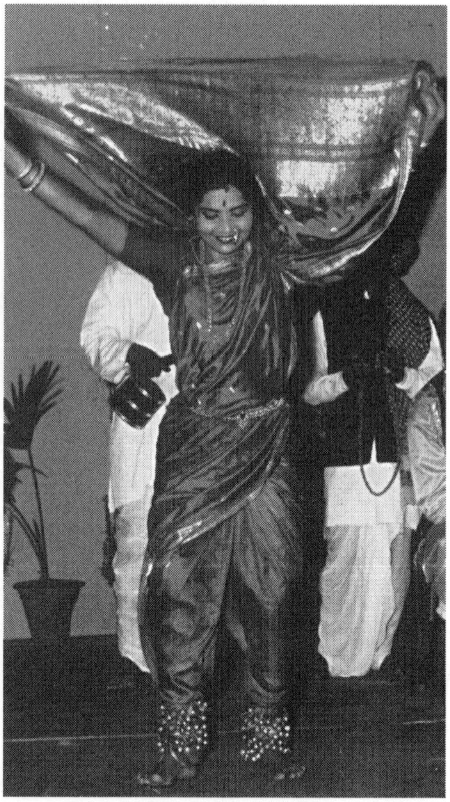

25. Tamasha, Maharashtra. Photo: SNA, New Delhi.

but those who are for stylized theatre, say that a theatre should be theatrical, because that is its character.

All these language theatre forms are basically arena theatres. They will appear incongruous on a proscenium stage. Some forms of like Mach of Madhya Pradesh erect a two- or three-tiered stage and simultaneous acting may be presented in two tiers. The Mach stage is also not like a proscenium stage.

Although our traditional language theatre forms as per their original style are aesthetically so satisfying, it is unfortunate that quite a few forms like Jatra of Bengal and Orissa, Nautanki of Uttar Pradesh is much influenced by the commercial films and as a result, losing much of its aesthetic appeal. They are imitating commercial films obviously for popular appeal. Unless they get a sizeable clientele who will dislike the cheap elements of commercial films, they will go on deteriorating and totally lose their delectable aesthetic character.

Jatra

Jatra literally means 'journey'. In the formative stage of this traditional folk theatre of Orissa, Jatra was a kind of processional theatre. This kind of rudimentary Jatra still survives in Puri and associated with religious ceremony is now performed every year at the time of Ramnavami. Locally it is called Sahi Jatra. In this processional theatre no dialogue is used. Masked actors represent various well-known epic characters and while in musical procession, with stylized gait, they depict through simple gestures a few selected and well-known episodes from the *Ramayana*. Since a procession is a kind of journey, it was named Jatra. From this processional theatre developed a kind of arena theatre which also bore the same name. In the sixteenth century, the popular *Lakshmi Purana* of Balarama Das was staged as an arena theatre.

J.C. Mathur and other scholars are of the opinion that around the twelfth century a kind of *uparoopaka* evolved which was called *sangeetaka*. According to them, the famous *Geetagovinda* of Jayadeva was categorically written for a *sangeetaka* presentation. The *sangeetaka* kind of *uparoopaka* was dominated by song and dance. The arena theatre Jatra had *sangeetaka* assists model.

Around the eighteenth century, some devout Vaishnavas originated *raas* (in colloquial Oriya also called *rahas*) groups and presented an Oriya version of *sangeetaka*, drawing exclusively upon the Krishna legend for their plays. This was in the same line of Krishna Jatras of Vrindavan and Mathura. In the third and fourth decades of the twentieth century a devout Vaishnava named Mohana Sundara Deva Goswami had an excellent *raas* group. The well-known Odissi dance *guru*, Kelucharan Mohapatra, was initially in this group. The *raas* was a kind of musical dance drama which used classical Odissi dance and music. The Jatra of Orissa has been much influenced by the *raas* in which dance and music dominate and which is more operatic than the Jatra of West Bengal.

Jatra is basically an actor-based theatre. All the actors in the traditional Jatra were men. Now, however some professional Jatra groups have actresses to play the female roles. A Jatra actor has to be a versatile performer, because he has to sing, dance and do stylized mime. The dialogues are either sung or delivered in a kind of recitative manner. Of course, the dialogues of the humorous sequences are delivered in plain prose. Earlier, most of the Jatra plays were mythological. Later all kinds of themes were admitted. Jatra is basically a stylized theatre. Therefore, melodramatic elements and stylized theatricality are its strong points. Realism is making gradual inroads into it via commercial movies and instead of enhancing the appeal it is robbing it of much of its theatrical vigour.

The arena for the presentation of Jatra performance may be on the level ground, but often it is a slightly raised platform. The audience sits on three sides of the arena. Often the audience sits on all four sides and the actors move in such a way that no side can be called as the front side of the arena.

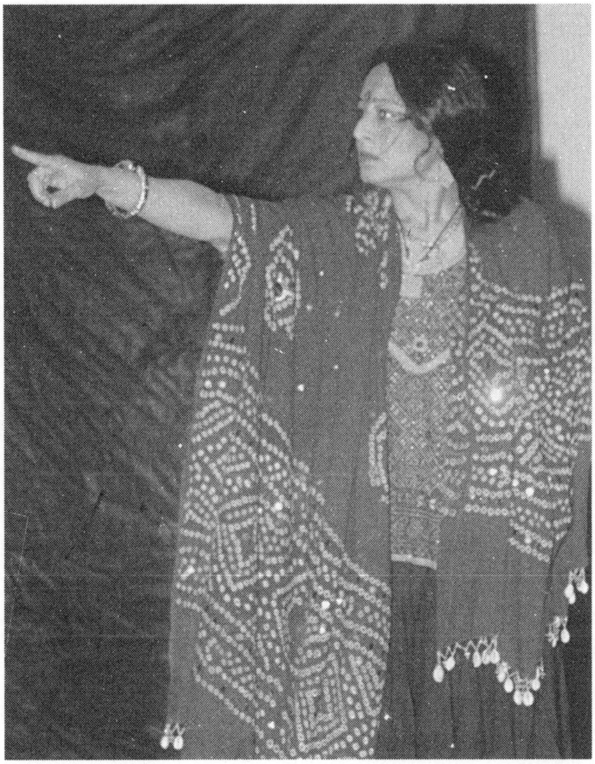

26. Ruma Bose, an amature stage performer of Delhi performing in a Bengali drama.

A 4 feet to 5 feet wide gangway, called *puspapatha*, literally the 'road of flowers', joins the arena with the green room. The gangway not only serves the function of entrance for the actors, but at times becomes an extended part of the acting area, especially when the stock character, *niyati*, meaning the destiny punctuates the dramatic sequences. The role of the *niyati* in a Jatra play is interesting. Invariably whatever the *niyati* says is in the form of a song. The *niyati* represents different things at different sequences: inner voice of the character when he/she is contemplating something, conscience, divine warning or fate.

In olden days the music of Jatra was traditional Odissi or folk, but towards the late part of the nineteenth century, Hindustani classical music became popular in Orissa. The various *ragas* like *Yaman*, *Bharat Kedar*, *Khamaj*, *Piloo*, *Kafi* and so on were taken up by the music composers of the Jatra theatre, and the *Thumri* style of singing influenced them a lot. As a result a distinctive type of Jatra music emerged. Also musical instruments like the harmonium, violin, trumpet and *tabla* almost completely replaced the indigenous instruments like *mardal* (Odissi *pakhawaj*), *mridanga*, *veena*, and flute. As a result, Jatra music became louder but highly popular. In the 1930s and 1940s when film songs had not spread their magic, the Jatra songs were quite popular with the masses. Nowadays the Jatra music is totally influenced by Hindi film music.

The stock character *sutradhar*, who introduces the play, now rarely appears. Another age-old stock character *dwari* (gatekeeper) or *bankuli bandi* (crooked stick) has been totally done away with. Although a minor character, the *dwari* used to add a good deal of humour with his typical stylized gait and humorous song/dialogue. Certain actors used to specialize in this character.

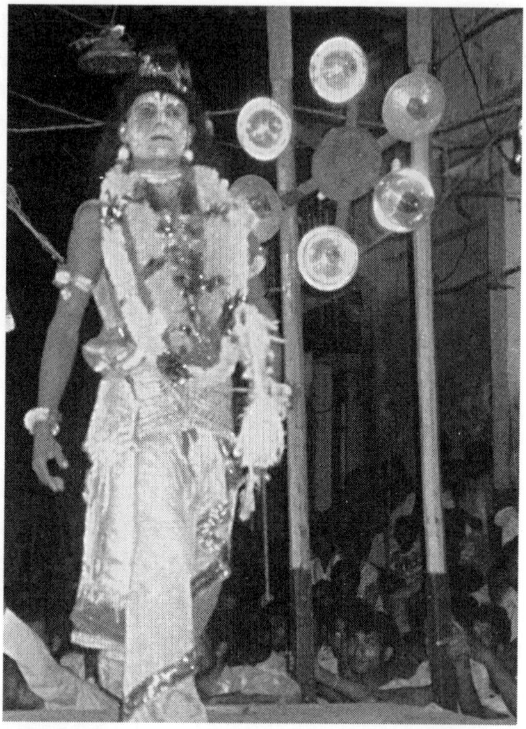

27. A performer performing the role of Rama on a wooden stage. Sakleswara Jatra Group, Nimapadara, Ganjam, Orissa. Photo: Dillip Tripathy.

There were quite a few palywrights for the Jatra theatre among whom Vaishnava Pani was the most powerful and popular. Now, of course, his plays are seldom presented by the professional groups.

Traditionally, before the Jatra proper begins, a typical tune is played by the orchestra. It is both a prelude (*poorva-ranga*) and a kind of announcement for the prospective audience that the play is about to start. After the orchestral flourish, a *gotipua* (a teenage boy dressed as a girl dancer) performs Odissi as curtain raiser. Although the dance is in Odissi style, it is more for the popular appeal than adhering to classical sophistication. After these preliminaries the play proper begins. The only prop used in Jatra is a chair. According to the dramatic situation, it can be a throne, a hiding place or a bathing *ghat*.

Although the professional Jatra groups have drifted away much from the tradition, some serious amateurs, at times, present old plays adhering strictly to the tradition and aesthetic considerations. Some of the modern Oriya directors are adopting some of the interesting presentational techniques of the Jatra theatre.

Daskathia

This is a fascinating form of ballad singing that admirably blends elements of theatre, music, wit and humour. It is, however, not as sophisticated as the other ballad singing tradition known as *pala*. *Daskathia* requires only two singer actors for the performance, the duration of which may be from around two hours to eight hours, that is, the whole night, depending upon the audience and the theme of the ballad. The main singer is called *gayaka*. He is assisted by the *palia*. Both of them play a kind of castanet called *daskathi* from which the form has derived its name. The *gayaka* plays bigger and different castanets, which is called *ramtali*. The *gayaka* plays it sparingly. It is the *palia* who is an expert in playing the smaller pair of castanets called *daskathi*. He punctuates the performance with percussion music of highly complex and fascinating rhythmic passages. He also punctuates with passages of wit and humour that enhance the appeal of the performance. Thus the importance of the *palia* is no less than that of the main singer. The *gayaka* must have very good voice, because it is he who sings the entire ballad and the *palia* echoes only the last one or two words of the sung line.

The singing style is more or less, in accordance with the *chhanda* form of Odissi classical music. The themes of the ballads are usually drawn from the vast body of Indian mythological literature, especially those which have Oriya versions. Invariably the *gayaka* himself composes the ballad in verse form, taking interesting episodes from the mythology. The *gayaka* not only sings but explains and elaborates in impromptu prose. He wears a costume that is similar to what the erstwhile rulers wore on formal occasions.

In *daskathia* the vocal music of the *gayaka* is accompanied by the percussion music of the castanets. No other musical instrument is used in this form of ballad singing.

Although *daskathia* originated in the southern part of Orissa, especially in the district of Ganjam, it has now spread to the other parts. But *daskathia* singers are still mostly found in Ganjam.

Pala

This is a unique form of ballad singing that aesthetically blends elements of theatre, classical Odissi music and highly sophisticated Oriya and Sanskrit poetry, wit and humour. It is more sophisticated than the other ballad singing tradition known as *daskathia*. Usually, there are six to seven perfomers in a group of *pala* singers. It cannot be traditionally presented with less than four performers. The leading singer is called *gana* (also *gayaka*), the percussionist is called *hana* who plays a two faced drum called *mridanga*, and two to five associate singers called *palias* of which the leading one is called *shreepalia*. The ordinary *palias* play large cymbals called *kartaal*.

Pala is presented in three ways: in the *baithaki pala*, all the performers sit on the ground throughout, in the *thia pala*, which is more popular and aesthetically more satisfying the performers stand while performing. The *badi pala* is a kind of *thia pala* in which there are two groups which vie with each other for excellence in performance. The last kind is the most entertaining, as there is an element of competition.

A loud percussion ensemble comprising the drum and the large cymbals, precedes the singing. In this *gana*, the leading singer does not participate. The purpose of the percussion ensemble is twofold, to let the prospective audience know that the *pala* is going to be presented soon and the other is to serve as aesthetic prelude (*poorva-ranga*). In the rural areas, the audience come to the performance after dinner. Therefore, it begins usually around 8.30 to 9 p.m.

At the end of the musical prelude, the *gana* enters the arena. Usually it is on level ground, over which a large cotton carpet is spread. The leading singer holds a flywhisk, called *chaamar*, in his hands, which is use in different ways at different times. He begins with an invocation eulogizing the presiding deity. Traditionally the *pala* is associated with the worship of Satyapeer, a saint accepted by both Hindus and Muslims. This trend can be traced back to the Mughal period when there was conscious effort to bring about amity between the two religious faiths. After the innovation the *pala* proper begins. As in *daskathia*, so also in *pala*, the ballad is structured by the *gana* himself, but the style of structuring differs. The major portion of the *pala* ballad is in stanzas of highly ornate Oriya poems written by eminent poets between the seventeenth century and the fourth decade of the twentieth century. The poems and *kavyas* (long narrative poems) written during this period were meant not only to be read but also to be sung in the *chhanda* styles of various kinds. The *gana* while structuring a particular *pala* ballad, follows the same pattern as that of the classical Oriya *kavyas*. A *kavya* in its initial phase poetically narrates the birth of the hero and the heroine. Different cantos describe their growing up through the phases of infancy, adolescence and youth. They meet and fall in love. Finally they marry. One or more cantos describe the beauty of the hero and especially the heroine in each phase of their growing up. The description of the beauty of the heroine from head to toe in her youthful phase is given in great detail with wonderful similies.

The *pala* ballad has the same structure. The descriptions of the various aspects of her/his beauty is not written by the *gana* but is taken directly from the *kavyas* of different poets. For instance, the *pala* writer wants to describe the beauty of the eyes of a youhtful heroine. He can take his pick of relevant stanzas from various *kavyas* written either in Oriya or Sanskrit and attribute them all to the heroine of the *pala*. This borrowing from various poets may go on for hours. The *gana* not only sings these stanzas in appropriate *chhanda* style, but also explains the meaning of the highly ornate lines in simple language. Thus through the *pala* sophisticated poetry was being popularized among common people. If the *gana* is not talented enough to structure a *pala* ballad, he may requisition the services of a suitable literary person to structure it for him. But he has to have an extraordinary memory to remember the countless stanzas and a high degree of literary sensibility so that he can properly explain the meaning as well as the poetic merit to the common people. The singer who agrees to participate in a *badi pala* has indeed a phenomenal memory and ready wit, because the other singer may challenge him on any aspect.

The *gana* is also an excellent actor. While singing or explaining he brings in dramatic acting to heighten the appeal. He then uses his flywhisk as different properties. At one time if it is used as the thunderbolt of Indra, another time it may delineate the lyrical movement of waves or the contour of a graceful creeper. He usually wears a costume similar to the formal dress of the erstwhile nobility. The others in the group wear a kind of costume which is not so splendid.

The role of the *palias* is more or less choral. They sing the refrain of the song together with the *gana* and echo the last few words of the other sung lines. The role of the *shree-palia* is of great importance in the performance as it is he who frequently interacts with the *gana* and punctuates the performance with wit and humour.

It is unfortunate that this unique, fascinating and dignified tradition of performing art is gradually disappearing because the people are so addicted to the popular mass media. The number of people, who would now prefer a *pala* performance to a film or a television serial is very very small. To be a good *gana* besides multifaceted talent, one has to devote years to study and practice. It has to be a fulltime job. If one is not assured that the earning from this profession can make a decent living, who will be tempted to master this difficult art? The last great *ganas* were Harinath and Niranjan. They were in great demand till the early 1950s. The demand grew less and less, but there were sporadic *pala* performances till the mid 1960s. Both have passed away. No one else has come up with even a fraction of their talent and excellence. These groups who perform *pala* now are not even a shadow of the real art. They are at best amateurs, far from the excellence of a professional *pala* singer.

Prahlada Nataka

This is a highly stylized theatre prevalent in the Ganjam district of southern Orissa. The tradition is not very old. Towards the later part of the nineteenth century, Raja Ramakrushna Chhotaraya, an Oriya feudatory ruler of Jalantar state, now annexed to Srikakulam district of Andhra Pradesh, conceived the first performatory form of Prahlada Nataka.

The first play was written by Gopinath Parichha, a poet and playwright who received generous patronage from the ruler. As a gesture of gratitude the playwright not only dedicated the work to the ruler but also ascribed its authorship to him. Within a few years of its birth, Prahlada Nataka became so popular that the rulers of neighbouring princely states were inspired to write or to commission other versions of Prahlada Nataka. No matter which version, the plot remains the same, based on the myth of Narasimha *avatar*, the man-lion incarnation of Vishnu.

The similarities of make-up and costume suggest that it was inspired by Therukoothu of Tamil Nadu and the Veethi Natakam of Andhra Pradesh but the performance style is closer to the Jatra of Orissa.

Prahlada Nataka has only one play in its repertoire. It is an arena theatre, presented in the open air and on level ground, but a must for the performance is a five or six tiered wooden platform, some 6-feet high. The top of the platform has an area of about 6 × 4 feet, on which is placed the throne of Hiranyakashipu, the demon whom the man-lion incarnation of Vishnu kills at the end. The platform is usually collapsible and easily erected and dismantled. An area of about 30 square feet is the acting area that is enclosed by ropes in front of the platform. To the left, about 20 feet from the platform, is a hollow structure representing the pillar Hiranyakashipu smote. The accompanying musicians take their places to the right of the acting area, close to the platform. The orchestra usually comprises three instruments: a harmonium, a two-faced drum called *mardal*, and *gini* (a pair of small cymbals). A few groups have now started using violin and trumpet, adding a touch of glamour but they actually enhance the aesthetic appeal of the music.

Music is the life breath of Prahlada Nataka. It not only provides the base but also determines the dramatic structure. Both vocal and instrumental music at appropriate places intensify the dramatic effect. Dialogues winged with music take the emotive intent further than realistic delivery. Prahlada

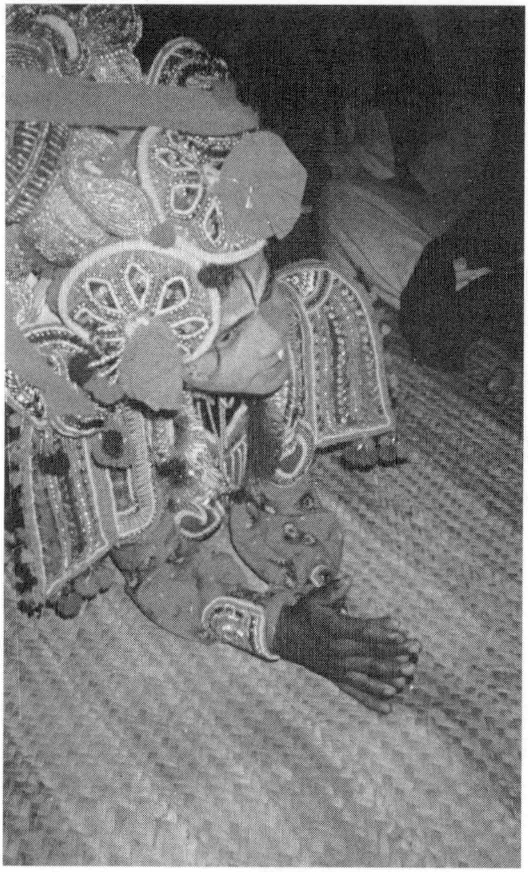

28. A nine years old boy performing the role of Prahlada. Photo: Dillip Tripathy.

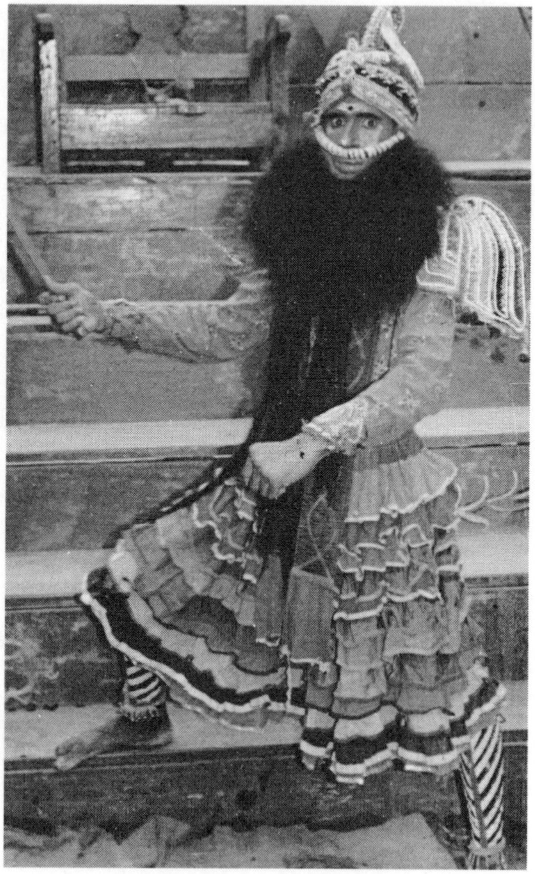

29. Hiranyakashipu of Prahlada Nataka with full costumes near the wooden altar. Photo: Dillip Tripathy.

Nataka draws heavily upon the traditional Odissi music that has a distinctive character of its own. Since music dominates Prahlada Nataka, the director (also the conductor) must be a good vocalist who has to memorize all the songs of the play. More often than not, the director himself acts as the leading vocalist called *gahaka*, derived from the Sanskrit word *gayaka* that means a singer. The *gayaka* is not the leader of the chorus, but he acts also as the interpreter, commentator, and the conductor of the orchestra. Although usually he does not wear makeup or costume, he has specific songs and dialogues. He sings eulogies of deities, narrates events preceding a dramatic situation, just before it is presented and

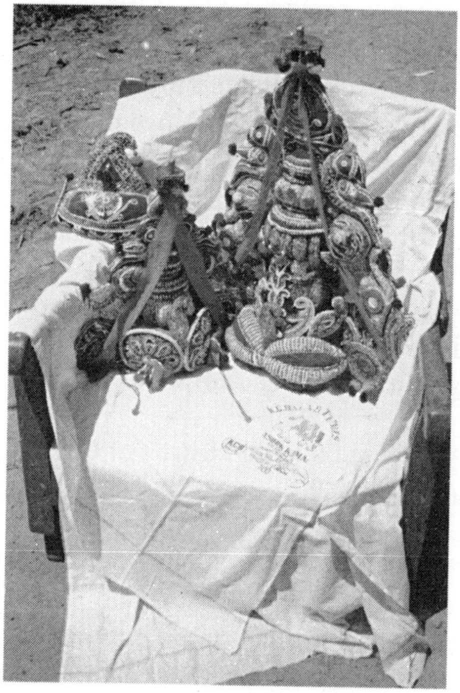

30. Headgears of Prahlada Nataka.
Photo: Dillip Tripathy.

also events pertinent to the plot but not enacted. At times, it is the *gayaka* who speaks the asides of a character and comments on his or her mood and thoughts. He is entrusted with the responsibility of explaining to lay spectators the cryptic, pithy dialogues. The role of this *gayaka* somewhat similar to that of a *sutradhar* of Sanskrit plays.

Although songs predominate there are also long prose passages, besides prose dialogues linking the sung passages. The role of Hiranyakashipu the demon is the most demanding. The way he goes up and down the tiered platform with vigorous dance like movements is indeed a treat for the eyes. A professional actor who excels in this role is at times hired by more than one group. Though Narasimha appears only in the last climatic scene and is seen on stage for only about a quarter of an hour, his again is a difficult role. The actor playing Narasimha fasts on the day of the performance. Putting on the lion mask and simulated claws, he stands amazingly transformed. It is said that years ago an actor playing the role had such complete with it, that he killed the one playing Hiranyakashipu. Apocryphal or true, the custom exists of tying a rope around the waist of Narasimha, the rope held by two or three stage hands who must avert a killing should the spirt of Narasimha take charge. The choice of an actor for the role is made with much care. In some villages such as Bokagaon near Chhatrapur the mask is worshipped in a temple and is believed to have divine powers.

Hiranyakashipu's face is painted bright red. His moustache is made of thick ropes of black thread twined with golden threads of *zari* and runs across the full expanse of the cheeks down to the nape of the neck where it is tied in a knot. Both Hiranyakashipu and Prahlada wear magnificently crafted headgear and colourful skirts. The major male characters were shoulder decorations. Apart from the female and the minor characters, all are costumed in such an exaggerated manner that they seem masked head to foot. In keeping with the stylizes makeup and costume, the acting is choreographic in character, with a high dose of song and dance.

Prahlada Nataka is so popular in the district of Ganjam that there are now more than thirty groups. All the groups are not equally good. But to watch the performance of Prahlada Nataka presented by a really good group is an unforgettable experience: tuneful music, dramatic dance, stylized mime, poetry, spectacle, colourful costumes and sumptuous decorations. All combine to induce a state of consciouness between wakefulness and dreaming. Refusing the 'trip', the literal-minded are likely to be bored at the end of the show.

The Chhau Dances

CHHAU IS A GENERIC name. In a contiguous area comprising north and west of Orissa, south of Bihar, and south-west of West Bengal, more than a dozen differing styles of dances are prevalent, which are called Chhau. Of these varying styles of Chhau, three are most representative and they are now called after the place of their prevalence. They are Mayurbhanj Chhau, Seraikela Chhau, and Purulia Chhau. While Mayurbhanj is in Orissa, Seraikela is now in Bihar and Purulia is in West Bengal, almost all the dancers are Oriya-speaking. The Mayurbhanj and Seraikela styles of Chhau are more evolved and sophisticated than Purulia Chhau, because the former were in princely states and their rulers extended enthusiastic patronage to the development of these dance styles. Like any classical style of dance, the two styles have a well-structured grammar of their own. Purulia Chhau, although not so evolved, is powerfully theatrical. Chhau is a unique form of dance in the sense that it admirably blends elements of classical, folk, and tribal dances. The principal difference between these three styles of Chhau is in the use of masks. While Seraikela and Purulia use masks, Mayurbhanj does not.

Although the dancers of all three styles of Chhau practice throughout the year: except during the rains, they formally present their performance to the audience on the last day or two of the month of *Chaitra* (March-April). Actually, the performance of these dances is an integral part of Chaitra Parva, the festival that both tribal and non-tribal communities celebrate to bid good-bye to the Indian year. Many other rituals are also performed as part of this festival, which are loosely associated with the dance presentation.

Another aspect that is common to all the styles of Chhau is the musical accompaniment. A Chhau orchestra must have one or more *dhols*, the barrel shaped drums with two faces, *dhumsa* or *dhak*, a huge bowl-shaped drum with one face, and *mahuri*, a woodwind instrument like the *shehnai* blown through a double reed. The musical styles of all three Chhau forms are also very similar.

All three Chhau styles have an unmistakably martial strain. Mayurbhanj Chhau emerged from a martial dance called *ruk-mar-nacha* that means the dance of defence and attack. Seraikela Chhau too, in its formative stage, was known as *phari-khanda-khela* meaning the play of shield and sword. In Purulia Chhau, almost all the dance numbers follow the conventional pattern of build-up in three stages: the encounter, the challenge, and the combat, culminating in the victory of the forces representing the good. Therefore, it is logical to surmise that Chhau dances evolved out of martial practices.

The other common similarity is the stylized leg extensions. In all the styles of Chhau dances the legs are more eloquent than the hands, may be because during the formative period the Chhau dancers were holding shields and weapons in their hands. A number of fascinatingly stylized basic steps and gaits are the foundation of all Chhau, with stylistic variations.

The element of theatre is pronounced in Chhau. Each dance number tells a story usually drawn from Puranic literature like the *Ramayana*, the *Mahabharata*, the *Bhagavata Purana* and so on. In the enactment, however, there is practically no verbal content. It is through stylized mimetic dance movements that the dancers tell the story. Therefore, Chhau is a kind of non-verbal theatre somewhat like Western ballet.

Mayurbhanj Chhau: This style of Chhau dance does not use any mask. Therefore, it sparkles with fascinating choreography, especially in group numbers, and with broad dance movements.

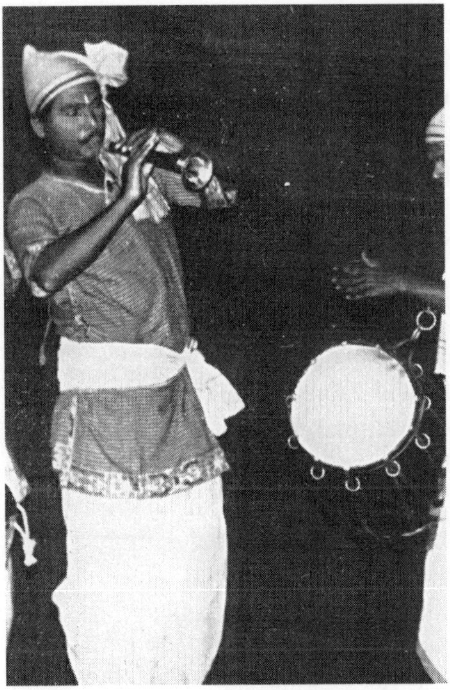

31. The archestra of Mayurbhanj Chhau. Photo: SNA, New Delhi.

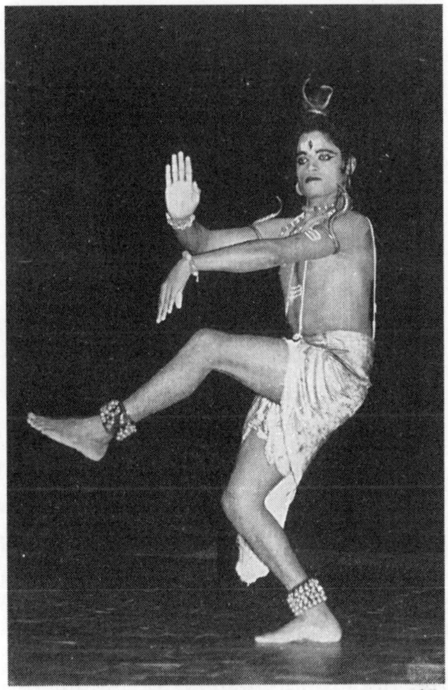

32. Sadasiva Pradhan performing Shiva *Tandav*, Mayurbhanj Chhau. Photo: SNA, New Delhi.

It evolved out of two forms of dance. One is a form of folk dance called *amdalia jamdalia nacha*, meaning the dance with branches of mango and *jamun*. The dance is so named because the dancers decorate themselves with small branches of mango and *jamun*. The other dance is known as *paikali*. In Oriya, *paika* means a soldier. *Paikali* therefore means the 'art of soldiers'. It is a form of martial dance. Each of the dancers performs holding a shield in the left and a sword in the right hand. These two dance forms still survive in a few very remote villages in Orissa. The leg extensions of the two dances are similar to that of Chhau dances. The musical instruments used in these dances too are exactly those used in Mayurbhanj Chhau. They are: *dhol*, a barrel-shaped drum with two faces *dhumsa*, a huge bowl-shaped drum with one face; *chadchadi*, a short cylindrical drum with two faces but played only on one face with two lean sticks; and *mahuri*, a woodwind instrument like the *shahnai* blown through a double reed. In the *paikali* dance the *ruk-mar-nacha*, that is, the dance of defence and attack, is an important part. It is also there in the repertory of Mayurbhanj Chhau, though performed in a much sophisticated way with fascinating choreography. One can see the presentation of Mayurbhanj Chhau as a part of Chaitra Parva at Baripada, the headquarters of Mayurbhanj district, every year on the last three days of the month of *Chaitra*, corresponding to 10, 11 and 12 April.

Mayurbhanj was an erstwhile princely state, whose rulers extended enthusiastic patronage to the dance. As a result, Mayurbhanj Chhau became more and more sophisticated and developed a well-structured grammar of dance movements. The basic units of dance phrases are called *tapka* and *ufli*. While the six kinds of *tapkas* are stylized gaits, the *uflis* are stylized leg extensions. It is interesting that a number of *uflis* have been inspired by the daily chores of the Oriya housewife. For instance, out of the 36 kinds of *ufli*, a few are: *basana maja* (cleaning utensils), *chhuncha dia* (mopping the floor), *haladi bata* (grinding turmeric on a stone slab), *sindoora pindha* (putting a dot of vermilion on the forehead) and so on. The images suggested by the names of such *uflis* are evoked by stylized movements of the leg. When performed, the feminine grace of the actual activities are transformed into elegant masculine dance movements.

The rich and extensive repertory of Mayurbhanj Chhau has three kinds of dance numbers: *phoot nacha* (solo dance), *jodi nacha* (duet dance) and *mela nacha* (group dance). The group numbers excel in choreography. In Mayurbhanj Chhau it is the visual poetry of movement alone that becomes stormy passion. The style is free, intense, affluent, and melodious, rendering the dance into a poem ablaze with her storms, volcanoes, rivers and lagoons.

Purulia Chhau: The Purulia style of Chhau uses masks like Seraikela Chhau, but with a function. Although Purulia Chhau masks are not as sophisticated as in the Seraikela style, they vibrate with a quality of earthiness and their function is to effectively stylize the mythological character and to enhance the theatricality of the presentation.

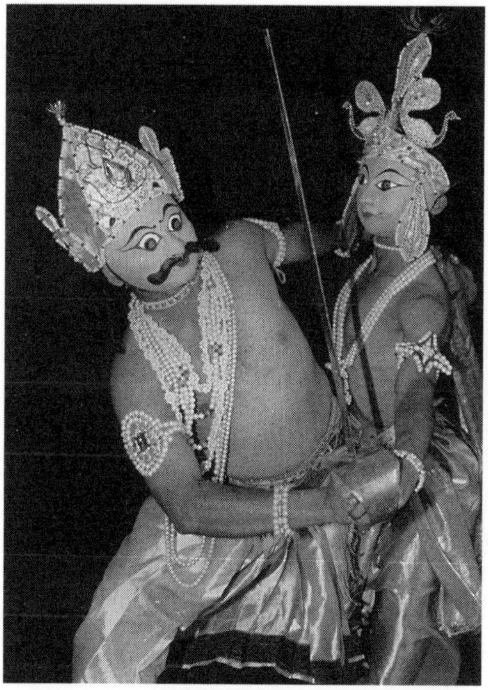

33. Sasadhar Acharya as Kansa and Sukanta Acharya as Krishna, performing the Seraikela Chhau. Photo: SNA, New Delhi.

The craftsman who prepares clay images of gods and goddesses in the Krishna Nagar style of clay-modelling, also makes masks for Purulia Chhau. The main centre of mask-making is Chorda, a village near Bagmundi town in the district of Purulia. The masks are made of papier mâché and integrated with towering and resplendent headgear. It is believed that the use of the mask in Purulia Chhau is an influence of *Gambhira*, a ritualistic dance tradition which is now rarely performed.

Purulia is in the state of West Bengal, that has a very powerful theatre tradition in Jatra. The dramatic vigour of Purulia Chhau and its resplendent costumes with ornate gold thread work bear the unmistakable influence of Jatra. Purulia was an estate under the administrative control of a *zamindar* (landlord) who did extend patronage to the dance style, but it was not as enthusiastic and participative as in the case of Seraikela. As a result, Purulia Chhau is not as evolved as the other two, and lacks an elaborate grammar of dance techniques. It has emphasis on dramatic vigour, rather than enhancement of the classical elements. A few different kinds of stylized walk, broad jumps and leaps in the air are all that a dancer has to master. But, even though Purulia Chhau does not have an elaborate dance grammar like Mayurbhanj and Seraikela, it is the most virile and dramatic of all Chhau styles.

All the dance numbers in the repertoire of Purulia Chhau are group compositions and they draw upon the *Ramayana* and the *Mahabharata* for their themes. The episode that each dance number depicts has three distinct phases of development. The first phase depicts the confrontation of a benevolent force with a malevolent force. The second phase depicts the fight between these two forces. In the third and the concluding phase, one of the forces is defeated. If the benevolent force is defeated, it is a tragedy, as in the dance number named *Abhimanyu Badh*. In most cases, however, the evil force is defeated as in a straight morality play.

Seraikela Chhau: In the Seraikela style of Chhau, the use of masks not only determined the line of its growth but remained its focal point even after the dance form crystalized fully. The mask is the quintessence of the character portrayed by the actor-dancer. Therefore, it needs very gifted artists to visualize the mask and to give shape and substance to it. Most of these masks require suitably ornate and stylized headgear to be complete. The headgear gives the mask a resplendent touch with coloured beads, artificial pearls and *zari* work and also artistically balances it when worn by the actor-dancer. The uniqueness of Seraikela Chhau is that these masks with neutralized expression become expressive during the course of the dance. The flow of movement and bodily expression, the positioning of the body in relation to the audience, contrive to express, at one time, great anguish and at another time, joy and happiness.

Masks used in Seraikela Chhau are of three types. One type represents mythological/historical/social characters, such as, Krishna, Radha, Jhansi ki Rani, Nabika (boatman) and such like. The second type is as interesting as it is poetic, since these masks represent abstract things

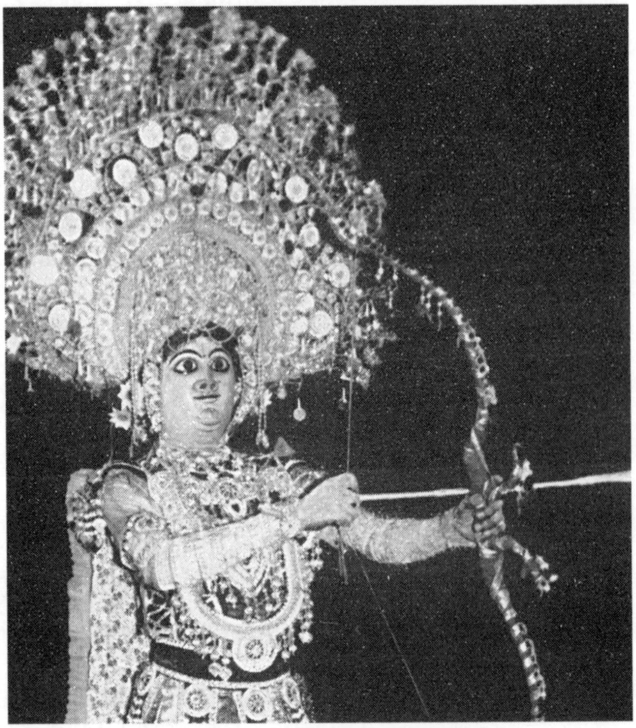

34. Satish Mahato as Kartikeya, Purulia Chhau. Photo: SNA, New Delhi.

conceived of as having human faces, such as *marumaya* (mirage), *ratri* (night) or *aleya*. The third type is also interesting as the masks represent animals and birds conceived of as having human face, such as, *mayura* (peacock), *hansa* (swan), *kuranga* (deer) and so on. The dancer does not imitate the bird or the animal, but depicts them as symbolically. For instance, the *mayura* symbolizes a narcissistic personality who is outwardly showy, but deep within stalks the shadow of an undefined disappointment.

Seraikela too was a princley state. The rulers and the nobility not only enthusiastically patronized the dance but actively participated in it. Prince Subhendra was a great dancer. When the Seraikela Chhau troupe visited Europe in the year 1937-8, he was acclaimed as a master performer. The dance critic of the *sketch* of 15 June 1938 says, 'The star dancer is Subhendra, and I am not going to compare him to Uday Shankar as they are both equally fine in their different way.' Again, almost all the dance numbers in the present repertoire of Seraikela Chhau have been choreographed by Bijoy Pratap who was the brother of the then ruler. Owing to the deep involvement of such talented members of the royal family, Seraikela Chhau accentuated the classical inherent in the dance form. The repertoire is therefore full of dance numbers with highly symbolic and poetic themes.

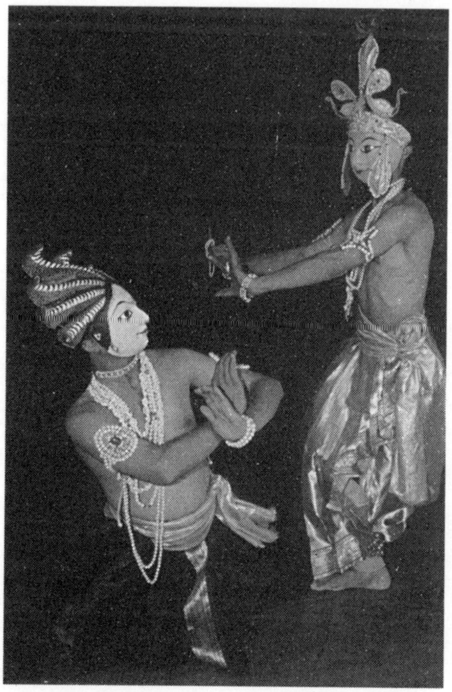

35. Sasadhar and Sukanta performing Seraikela Chhau. Photo: SNA, New Delhi.

Seraikela Chhau evolved out of the *pharikhanda khela* literally, 'the play of the shield and the sword'. It is a martial dance and is still prevalent in Seraikela. The basic units of dance phrases, called *chhali* and *uphlei* bear great similarity with the *topka* and *ufli* of Mayurbhanj Chhau. They are marked by their highly stylized leg extensions.

One can see the presentation of Seraikela Chhau as a part of Chaitra Parva festival every year on the last day of the month of *Chaitra*, corresponding to 12 April, at Seraikela, the sub-divisional headquarters of district Singhbhum, Bihar. A sensitive spectator watching the performance will experience how, with aesthetically crafted masks, Seraikela Chhau takes fantasy to the summit of poetry, where beauty is distilled from a world of magnificent dreams.

Shadow Theatre: The Ancient Movie

SHADOWS PRESENT objects in an unknown dimension. A shadow intentionally created to represent an object or a living being appears fascinating because of the inevitable stylized lineament. When such shadows move to delineate an event, the effect is at once mysterious and dramatic.

The shadow theatre also known as shadow play or shadow show is, in fact, a kind of puppetry. Flat puppet figures, usually made of leather, are lightly pressed on a translucent screen with a strong source of light behind. The audience sitting on the other side of the illuminated screen does not see the puppets but sees their shadows on the screen. The puppeteers who manipulate the figures place themselves in such a way that neither are they seen by the audience nor do their shadows fall on the screen.

Although it is a kind of puppetry, this is delightfully different from all other forms of theatre. One the human and puppet stages, a real world of three dimensional space is created, in which actors or articulated figures have direct contact with the audience. But in shadow theatre, the contact is always indirect, as the audience sits on the other side of the screen. Thus, spectators and actors separated by the light screen are placed as if in different rooms. The spectator is by himself and his feeling of isolation is heightened by the darkness all around. He does not directly experience the figures and the play, he only sees the image, in its projection. The light screen here is most important, as it filters and

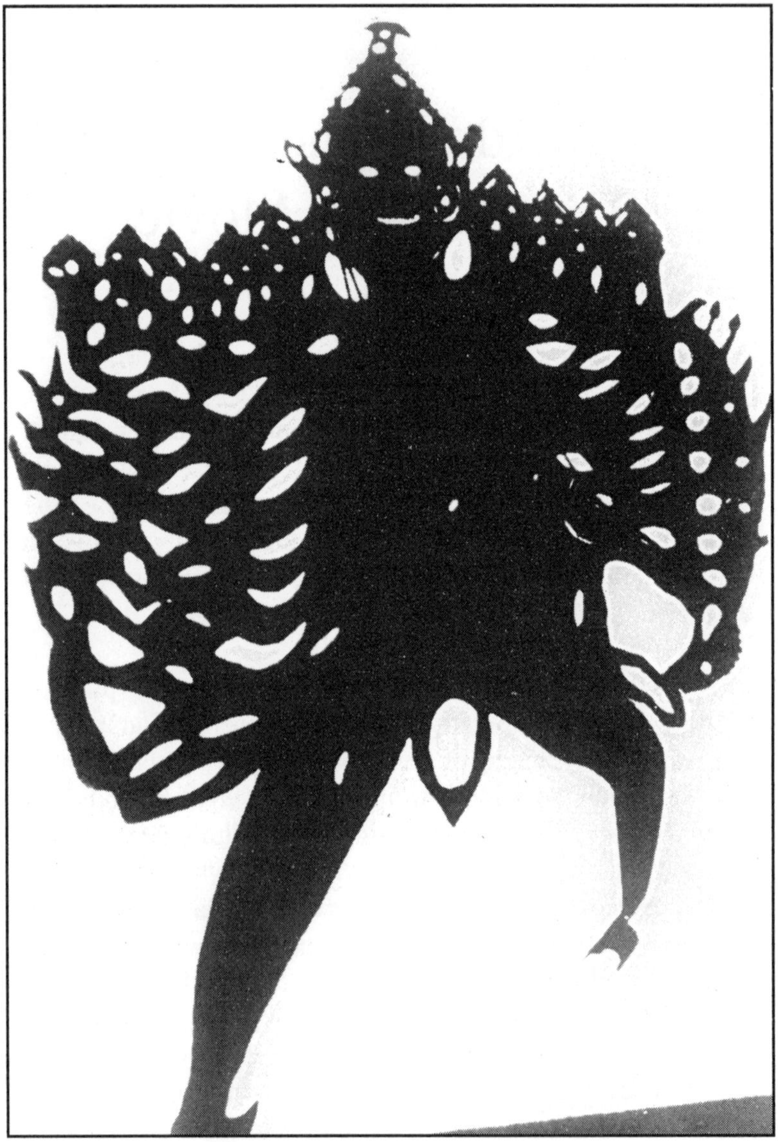

36. Ravana, Ravanchhaya shadow puppetry.
Photo: SNA, New Delhi.

modifies the image and modifies the action. On the 'inner' side of the screen, the actor (the manipulator) too is isolated. He presents a projection of his thoughts and expects the spectator to interpret and to re-assemble them into a new image. It is not the object in his hand but its image on the screen that decides his action. There are thoughts and ideas in his fantasy. He translates them into moving shadow pictures. In the mind of the audience these pictures are retranslated into happenings. This is what makes shadow theatre an exciting experience.

The term 'motion picture' applies more accurately to the shadow theatre. Because in cinema the pictures do not move but a sequence of consecutive pictures of objects, photographed in motion by specially designed cameras, is thrown on a screen by a projector in such a rapid succession as to give the illusion of natural movement. In shadow theatre the pictures *actually move*. Therefore, shadow theatre can be called as the most ancient form of the movie.

The tradition of shadow theatre not only originated in India, but reached a high degree of evolvement and sophistication. It is unfortunate that such a rich tradition has been languishing in remote rural areas for the last hundred or more years without patronage, without connoisseurship. Fortunately, six varying styles of traditional shadow theatre still survive, in the rural areas of Orissa, Maharashtra, Kerala, Tamil Nadu, Karnataka and Andhra Pradesh.

Among these six styles of traditional shadow theatre, while the Orissa, Maharashtra and Kerala styles throw black and white shadows on the screen, the Tamil Nadu, Karnataka and Andhra styles throw coloured shadows. A sensitive theatre-goer, to whom a stylized presentation gives much deeper and more intense dramatic experience than the realistic, will be thrilled to witness any of these styles of traditional shadow theatre. His reward is the form's dramatic vigour, for it can take drama to heights from beyond the reach of any live actor.

The traditional shadow shows have each a particular name in the language of the regions where they prevail. In Kerala, it is Thol Pava Koothu (Malayalam), in Tamil Nadu, Tholu Bommalatam (Tamil), in Karnataka, Togalu Gombeyatta (Kannada), and in Andhra Pradesh, Tholu Bommalata (Telugu). The literal meaning of them all is 'dance of the leather puppets'. The Maharashtrian shadow show is, however, called Chamdyacha Behulye meaning leather puppets. In this style the puppet figures are mostly non articulate and therefore perhaps, dance is not added to the name. The way Orissa shadow show has been named is interesting, in the sense that the usual pattern is not followed. It is called Ravanchhaya, meaning the shadw of Ravana. The three opaque styles, prevalent in Kerala, Maharashtra and Orissa that present their shadows in black and white, base their themes exclusively on the legend of Ram. Naturally it would have been more appropriate if the Orissa shadow show had been named Ramchhaya, but there is an interesting metaphysical reason for naming it otherwise. Ram is a dream and the word *devata*, deits is derived from the root *div* meaning to shine. Therefore, the literal meaning of the word *devata* is a shining being which cannot cast its own shadow. Besides, shadow is dependent on light. His physical shape may cast a shadow, but to join Ram's name with 'shadow' appeared incorrect.

Of all the differing styles of leather puppets, those of the Ravanchhaya, made of deer skin are the least sophisticated. They are made of a single piece of skin and have no joint limbs. The cutting and stencilling of the figures are done with an apparent naivete. Looking at them, one can never imagine their shadows will be wonderful, bold and dramatic. Although not articulated, they are manipulated with a kind of jigging and the technique never appears inadequate to a sensitive audience which has a taste not for gimmicks, but for subtleties.

The leather puppets of Maharashtra are, though mostly unarticulated, a shade more sophisticated than those of Ravanchhaya. The only living puppeteer of Pinguli village (Maharashtra) does not know how to prepare a new puppet figure. The ones he has are more than 150 years old. They are the smallest of the six styles of leather puppets. The parchment also is much thinner.

So far as the actual stencilling is concerned, the Kerala style puppets are unsurpassed. Filigree like chisel cuts on the leather wonderfully delineate the jewellery and the embroidered costume shows the puppet's character. Like Ravanchhaya puppets these figures also look drab, but their shadows are breath takingly beautiful and they show what enrichment a silhouette can have. Of the three styles of shadow theatre, that of Andhra Pradesh uses the largest figures ranging from 4 to 6 feet. These figures have also multiple jointed limbs and therefore, are the most mobile. In Karnataka, two kinds of leather puppets are used, a larger one resembling the Andhra puppet and the other, called *chikka*, which is small in size ranging from 1.5 to 2.5 feet. The *chikka* shadow presents highly decorative group scenes, each depicted in one figure. These group figures are brought on to the screen like freeze shots, to punctuate and intensify the dramatic effect. A few group figures like Ravana abducting Sita in *Pushpaka Vimana*, have joint parts to give partial articulation to the unarticulated figures.

The shadow theatre tradition of Tamil Nadu is on the verge of extinction. So far only one traditional puppeteer could be traced. He has a few old leather puppets beautifully coloured with vegetable dyes, but since making a leather puppet is quite expensive he had to resort to cheaper materials like cardboard, tissue and cellophane paper for the purpose. The art may be lost for ever if the clientele for it does not increase many times of what it is now. (Tamil Nadu has since seen a partial 'revival', with such folk forms being used by NGOs to spread social messages.)

Although the shadow theatre traditions are barely surviving, owing to the stagnation of patronage, for more than a few centuries, their quality of production has suffered a lot. Yet what survives, be it any of the styles discussed above, will offer many prize moments to a sensitive audience. Dramatic scenes, such as, Ram and Ravana fighting and their shadow arrows flashing across the screen like dark lightning, or Hanuman uprooting the shadow trees of the Ashok Vatika or setting fire to the golden city of Lanka, or Arjuna's arrow beheading a Kaurava stalwart, come out with such dramatic and lyrical beauty that it is inconceivable in any other form of theatre.

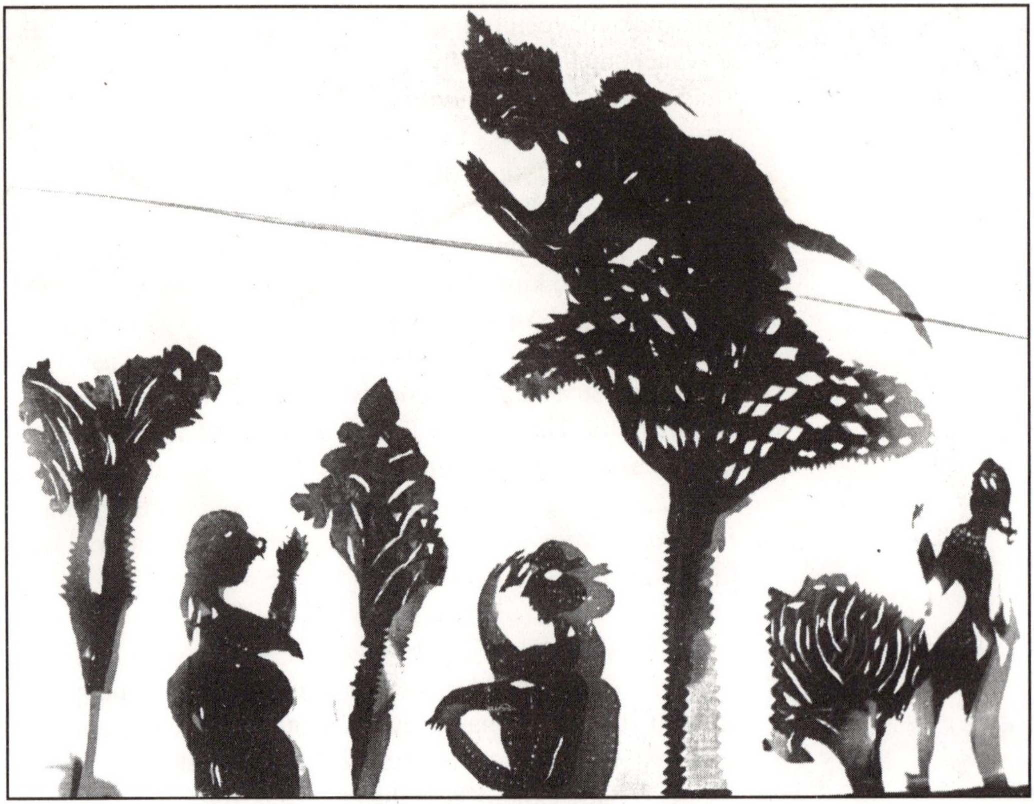

37. Hanuman in Ashok Vatika, Ravanchhaya shadow puppetry.
Photo: SNA, New Delhi.

It will be a great pity if such aesthetically rich and fascinating traditions die out because of utter negligence. Government patronage cannot make an art tradition live for ever, especially in a democratic set up. Again, it is the size of the clientele that has always decided the health of an art form. Unless the sensitive members of our society turn a part of their interest away from the intoxicating and glamourous media like movie, TV and video, and direct it towards the shadow theatre which is aesthetically far more satisfying, this tradition cannot be saved from the cruel hands of time.